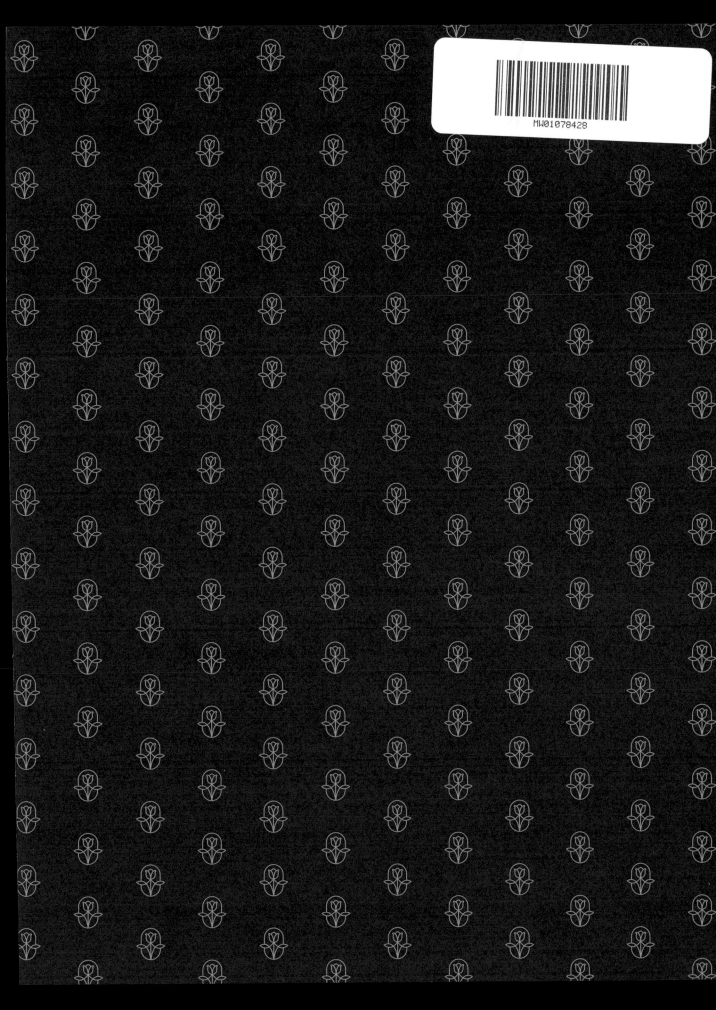

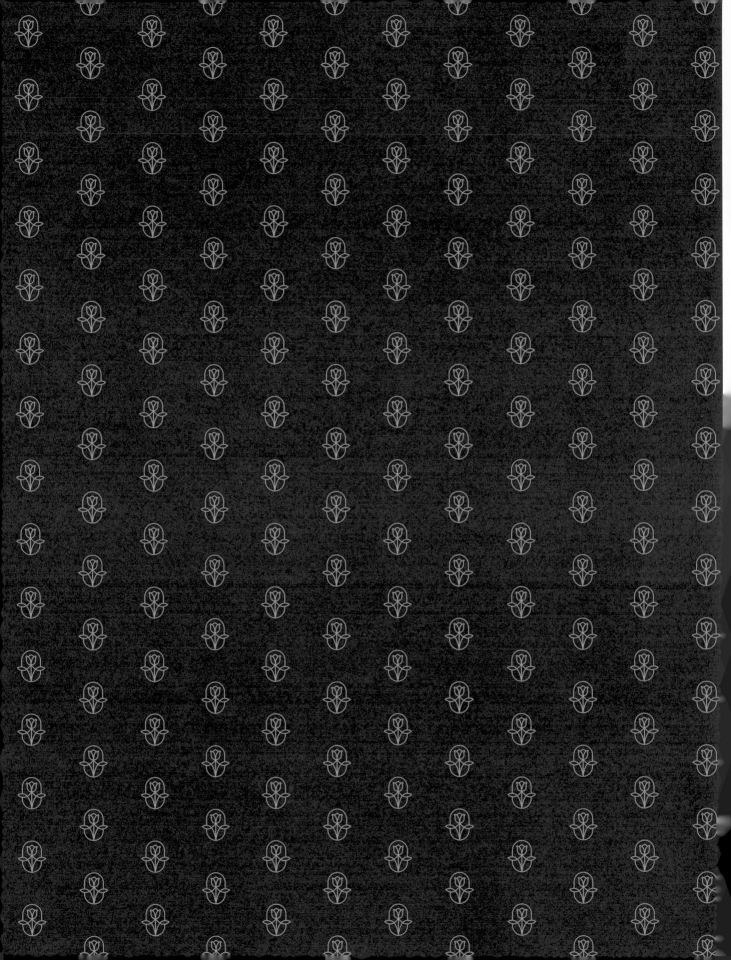

DAVID KIBBE'S
POWER OF STYLE

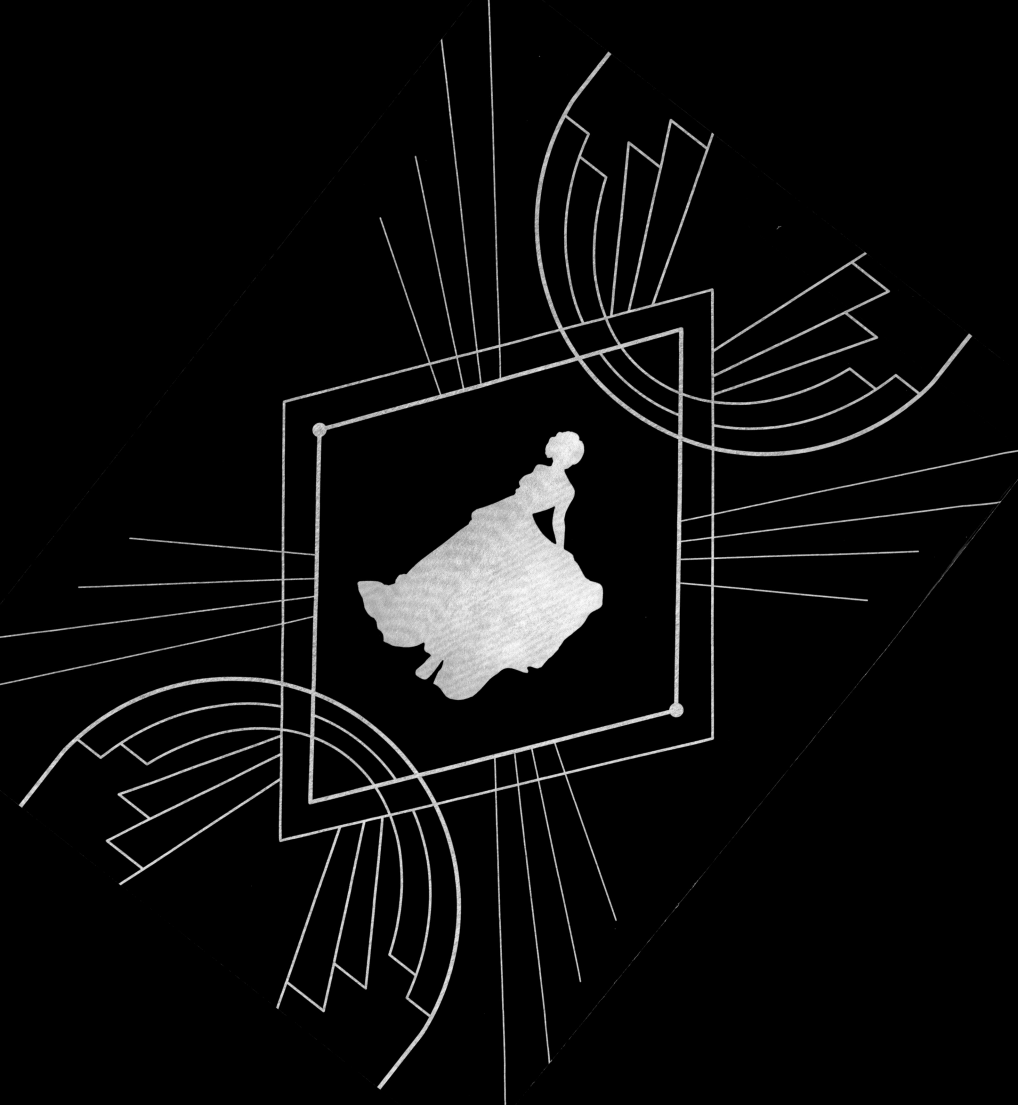

A NEW VISION OF BEAUTY

DAVID KIBBE'S POWER OF STYLE

A GUIDED JOURNEY TO HELP YOU DISCOVER YOUR AUTHENTIC STYLE

BY DAVID KIBBE

RODALE

NEW YORK

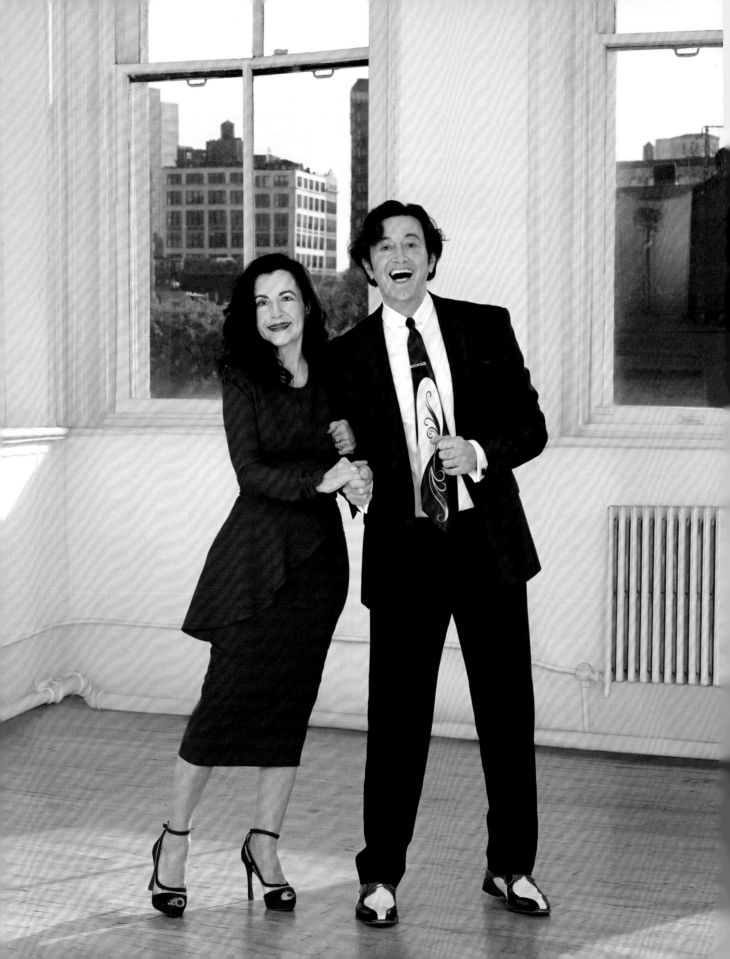

For Susan Slavin: wife, soulmate, eternal partner, and best friend, who constantly astounds me every day with the magnitude of her soul and the beauty of her spirit, with endless gratitude and infinite love.

FOREWORD

BY SUSAN SLAVIN

It started out with a prayer. I still weep with wonder when I think about it. . . .

Let me move ahead quite a bit. Several weeks ago, David asked me to write the foreword to this book. I was genuinely surprised! Aren't I way too close to him, this work, and every detail of the book to write anything the least bit objective?

So, I wrestled with the idea by myself for far too long. Finally, I decided to just ask David WHY he wanted me to do it. He said simply, *"Well, you're the ONLY one who could do this because you've been there since before the beginning, and you created everything with me."*

(I then realized that actually, I was kinda like Exhibit A, too!)

So, having been convinced, let me start by saying I really am proud to have the privilege of introducing you to what you are about to discover in these pages, as well as sharing a bit of the backstory of how it all came to be.

I will tell you right off, it's nothing short of a miracle that David's work has gotten to this point! But, truth be told, my whole life has been all about miracles—*believing* in them, following my dreams, listening to my heart and manifesting them. So a part of me is not surprised at all—just incredibly grateful.

Some of you may know David Kibbe as this guy who seems to have endless knowledge about our bodies and what to put on them. You may also think he's gotten to his status as a pop phenomenon overnight! The reality couldn't be further from the truth. . . .

A FATEFUL PROFESSIONAL ENCOUNTER

I was walking down a hallway talking intently about music with this young guy I had recently met. Out of the blue—without really looking at me—he blurted, "You know, you should wear RED!"

Wh-a-a-t?!! I reeled at his forwardness. Then my feelings started tumbling, one after the other. In the blink of an eye, I went from startled—to wary—to titillated—to intrigued—and then, to sudden relief. I could breathe. I got very calm. WOW! This guy who didn't know me, SAW me. And, oddly enough, I felt he CARED.

That guy was David Kibbe, and what he did for me in that instant, he had been doing his whole life. He could SEE and would CARE about everyone he ever met. And—he wanted to HELP.

So that laser vision and empathy and need to make things better for everybody were at the core of who he was. Not long after that, I realized he was all about LOVE, though he never spoke about that. . . .

But then something else occurred. We became inseparable. When I lost my glasses, I'd wear his.

When I looked down, we were always walking in exact step together. We saw the world with the same eyes and we moved in unison forward in our lives. And oh boy! I was enchanted by David.

Inevitably, we fell deeply and passionately in love with each other.

And we knew.

It was everlasting.

And the truth is, our love story is at the center of everything that is going to unfold in the following pages.

Which brings me to . . .

THE PRAYER

David had recently returned from acting in a national tour ending at the prestigious Kennedy Center in Washington, DC. It had been hard for us to be apart, and we had a joy-filled, tearful reunion. But soon I sensed a heavy sadness in him. Where was his usually ebullient personality? He was at that lull between jobs, waiting for his agent to call. But, somehow I felt it was way more than that.

I knew David to be a creative force to reckon with. He had already amassed impressive credentials as a star actor, and all-around bravura auteur after also having been a brilliant young classical pianist from an early age. Now however, his life seemed to be *on hold*.

What was wrong with this picture? It profoundly troubled me to feel his pain. Was there *anything* I could do?

I had an idea but wasn't sure how he would react. We were about to go to dinner, and I carefully asked if we could meditate together on his situation. He was wide open. Relief! So I suggested we sit facing each other, hold hands, close our eyes, and breathe.

"Dear God—and all the angels—please help David find a new way to use his great gifts in his daily life."

We sat in silence. We breathed. We knew something was coming.

Within one week almost to the day, the perfect new opportunity appeared! He felt he could juggle this with his acting career and decided to go all out for it. He started working as a beauty/style consultant. And the rest, as they say, is history. . . .

"THE HARDER HE WORKED, THE LUCKIER HE GOT"

That old adage could have been written for David! I had never known anyone with his kind of work ethic—or to move with such lightning speed.

One day soon thereafter, we were walking down the street and David was ruminating. He believed there needed to be something that had never existed before, a SYSTEM that crystallized his method of working with clients which would help everyone see themselves accurately. At the same time, it would also need to unleash their unique spirit. (I had learned David was not capable of an unoriginal thought!) I listened. His wheels were turning at full speed.

Well, this was the beginning of his creating a whole new *paradigm* for identifying people—his Image Identity system.

He began with one client at my living room table. That one client became two, ten, twenty, one hundred, and on and on, culminating into many thousands of clients who traveled from all over the world to work with him. My living room springboarded to a small studio, and then, a large atelier with twenty-one employees!

Out of his initial Image Identity concept, he wrote the bestselling *David Kibbe's Metamorphosis,* which led to him becoming an internationally known media personality, as well as a much-sought-after expert source for all things beauty and style—today's reigning image guru on social media.

And so it went. And so it goes. . . .

ANOTHER NEW BEGINNING

Now, here we are at this astonishing moment, about to give the baby to the world with the launching of this new, long-awaited second book! I have to admit I am pretty giddy with excitement imagining you reading and seeing it for the first time. My personal feeling is that what you are holding in your hands is a treasure unlike any other. A gift that keeps on giving.

If you were led to it seeking beauty and style guidance, I can assure you it will exceed your expectations. I can also promise you many giggles on a scintillating fun ride! As to the rest—well, let's just say I hope you will uncover it all for yourself. . . .

So, without further ado, I will finish this prelude and turn it over to David. But one last thing before I do. I'd like to end the same way I began—the way it all began: with a prayer.

However, this one is for you.

Wherever this book finds you in your life—whether it's on a dark night—or a brilliant sunny day . . .

May it lead you to your dearest dreams being realized, quixotic surprise and delight along your way. And above all—may MIRACLES appear beyond your imagining.

With love,
Susan

CONTENTS

INTRODUCTION

A WORD OF WELCOME

Dear Friend,

Hello and welcome to my world! We are about to begin a journey together that I hope will transform your life.

If you are an old friend returning, I am overjoyed to have you back. If this is your inaugural trip with me, I invite you to join with open arms.

This is a voyage through a land of self-discovery. Here you will learn many exciting eye-openers, *new concepts* that I am grateful to be the messenger of:

***BEAUTY COMES FROM INDIVIDUALITY.

***STYLE *EVOLVES* FROM IDENTITY.

***THERE ARE NO "FLAWS"—ONLY UNIQUE CHARACTERISTICS.

***YOU ARE EXACTLY WHO YOU ARE "SUPPOSED" TO BE.

***THERE IS ONLY ONE "YOU."

***YOU ARE A STAR—IT IS YOUR IRREFUTABLE BIRTHRIGHT.

These are but a few of the basic stopovers along our travels. We will take the time to explore all the who, what, whys, and hows of all these fundamentals, each of which is essential to achieve your transcendent metamorphosis.

These are the bedrocks my work is based upon. Every element of what we are about to explore comes from the application of these epiphanies.

So let me be your guide, your friend, your confidant, as we get ready to set sail. This is a journey of aspiration, fueled straight from the heart, centered in the soul.

And so, let me introduce to you *A BRAND-NEW VISION:*
LOVE-BASED BEAUTY.

Our destination: *your transformation.* My ultimate goal: *to give you your wings.*

A LITTLE ABOUT YOUR GUIDE . . .
AND THE ORIGINS OF OUR JOURNEY

Since we are going to be sharing this journey, filled with all your hopes, wishes, and dreams, and I am asking you to trust me to lead you down this pathway, I think it only fair you should know a little bit about your guide, as well as how I came to create what we are about to undergo together.

First, I am honored, humbled, and totally delighted to share this with you. This book has been years in the making. It's the compilation of a lifetime's work. Creating this original approach to style and guiding so many through this journey over decades has been my total joy. I grew up in a small town in Missouri, right in the center of what we were told was the Mason-Dixon Line. At the time, we were famous for having BOTH an uptown and a downtown—uptown was one side of the railroad tracks, downtown was the other!

While I loved so much of my little town, the people, and especially my family, I always was also a bit of a dreamer, and it's those very dreams that created what has become my life's work, and what I hope to share with you.

From the very beginning of my existence, I had three innate yearnings that lit my way (and not necessarily always in the same order): ART, BEAUTY, and METAPHYSICS.

ART has been my passion from day one and I feel grateful to have been blessed with many talents: music, drama, dance, fine art. These were my connection to life from my earliest age, and I feel fortunate to have achieved success, along with critical acclaim, as an adult in all these areas.

I certainly claim no credit for the talent, as these were gifts that were bestowed upon me from above. I am eternally thankful for these, but they were not of my doing.

What I do take responsibility for is the skill I developed. I have worked diligently every day of my life making the most of what I've been given. Whatever the medium, I always have had this need to master it, to the best of my ability.

Personally, I believe in always striving to be the best possible vehicle for whatever gifts we have been blessed with. For me, the end result of this quest is the total bliss that comes when we share our gifts with the world.

How exactly this relates to the way I created things here certainly has to start with my earliest love affair with the arts—the piano.

I was known as a child prodigy. Starting at age three, I could read music before I could read language. My first recital appearance was at age five. By my high school years, I was an award-winning competitor. Out of ten competitions, I had nine firsts, one second. (I gained more from the second place than any of the firsts.)

My teacher at this time was one of the "greats." I credit her with every success I've subsequently had in every area of my life. One of the most elemental lessons I learned from her and have poured into this work is that talent is wonderful, but it's the TECHNIQUE that takes our gifts and turns them into ART.

Passion requires a cultivated craft in order to manifest. When transformed into art, it has the power to change the world.

Style (as we will come to define it) is our PERSONAL ART. Our journey is all about how together, we will learn the craft to achieve this magical transformation!

What I also have discovered and hope to help you realize is that style must evolve as we, both as individuals and the world around us, evolve. Every day, from the beginning of my work, I have strived to refine and expand what we are about to undergo. I want us never to simply settle for maintaining a status quo when there is the chance to improve, clarify, and elevate.

BEAUTY was just a given. I saw it everywhere. I was lucky enough to have parents who made sure their children were exposed to all sorts of culture, and we lived in a glorious natural setting filled with leafy trees and fragrant gardens all throughout the area I grew up in.

But what occupied much of my earliest imagination involved the many women who surrounded me from toddler time on.

In my town, most of the women in my parents' circle were homemakers. The dads went to the office (mine was a beloved lawyer); the moms stayed home, raising the kids and keeping house. Despite their busy schedules, somehow the women always found time for socializing during the day.

Coffee at my mother's table was a daily occurrence. (My mother's name was Barbara.)

Neighbor: "Knock-knock, Bobbi, in the mood for a cuppa?"

Mother: "Door's open, come on in, pot's on the stove."

This was daily music to my five-year-old ears. This meant I was going to get to sit on a lap, give a kiss on the cheek, and ask my mother's friend, "Will you marry me?" I even had a standard line: "Will you wait for me to grow up?" (At one count early on I had sixteen fiancées.) Even my babysitters were sworn to my future matrimony!

To my young eyes, their lips were the most beautiful red you could imagine. Their hair was always perfectly coiffed, and they were always dressed to the nines. Each one was like a beautiful angel had floated into my world.

I have to admit, five-year-old me forged my still-prevalent vision of beauty. I have never met a woman I didn't see as completely beautiful. It's their very uniqueness that is so glorious.

BEAUTY makes our heart smile and brings forth joy from the soul. It emanates from deep inside us and radiates out to everyone with whom we come into contact. It is our heart's connection to each other, and our liaison to the heavens.

METAPHYSICS is and always was something I couldn't explain but simply knew. While it's taken many different forms throughout my life, it's always occupied my entire being. I've always been on a search for our deepest connections to life.

There's a story that was often told about me from when I was about five years old (it seems this was a seminal age!). It's said one day when there was company at my house, I came in, walking around the room with a pronounced limp. My mother had me take off my shoe, to reveal a wad of paper inside. When she asked me why it was there, I responded that it was a message to God, as we had learned in Sunday school you talked to God through your "sole."

Years later, as an adult, my wife and I worked with a brilliant healer who did amazing astrology charts. Part of her work was to explore our "soul's journey" and what it meant. When she got to this section on my chart, she simply said one thing and left it at that: "Some people study metaphysics—David, you ARE metaphysics!" I just move through life knowing there is more to us than what we traditionally accept as "reality," knowing *possibilities* are where our greatest truths can be found.

This is the awareness in me that drives the essential part of my philosophy of beauty, as well as what I understand the true power of style to be. It's embedded deep within me, at my core. It's more than just a belief. It's stuff I just know.

We each are lit from the same source that powers the universe. Each of our lights is unique, special, and essential.

To say we are stars is not simply a metaphor. It is the unequivocal truth. We have the power of this light at our fingertips when we understand our special and unique place and purpose.

STYLE is the way we each choose to lavish our light.

So, from the silly to the sublime, these are the seeds from which this journey we are about to share has sprung. I created the entire structure, with its unique approach to style, from my own perspectives, history, experience, and vision.

As we travel this journey together, it's so important to me that you realize I am your champion. I created this program with one purpose only: *to give you your freedom.* My goal is to release you from all boxes, chains, prejudices (from either within or without), and preconceptions.

I see you from one viewpoint: *your potential.* I just can't bear anyone settling for anything less than having the tools to fly as high as you dare!

OUR JOURNEY BEGINS

As we get ready to take off, I want to remind you of the essential element of our trip. THIS IS A GUIDED JOURNEY with a starting point and ending point, with every stopover along the way designed to lead to the next. The magic unfolds step by step, and untold treasures exist at every stop. I will be right with you at every point, helping you through each step as we move forward together. Your destination *emerges* as the result of our traveling the entire pathway.

There are two components to discovering the POWER OF YOUR STYLE:

1. **RECONCEIVE THE MEANING OF STYLE.**
   A New Vision of Love-Based Beauty

2. **THE NUTS & BOLTS OF STYLE.**
   Learning the Technique to Manifest Your Style

OUR DESTINATION: YOUR FREEDOM.

MY ULTIMATE GOAL: TO GIVE YOU YOUR WINGS!

PART

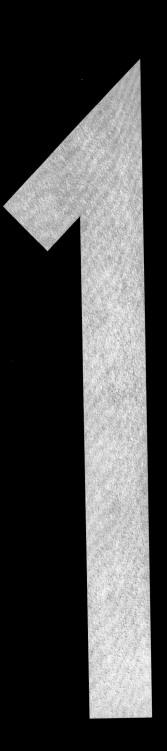

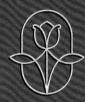

REDEFINING STYLE

THE NEW VISION

LOVE-BASED BEAUTY

> *There is only love or fear. . . . Every moment offers the choice to choose one or the other.*
>
> —ELISABETH KÜBLER-ROSS AND DAVID KESSLER

I firmly hold that, as one-of-a-kind beings, we all come to this planet created exactly as who we are supposed to be. If that's the case, then part of what makes us special is our physical being. *In other words, an unparalleled part of who we are is what we look like.*

I'm not suggesting that our outer self is all that we are. Of course it's not. Our "inside selves" have a vast range of qualities. We're not just one thing in there. We have a multitude of inner essences, and our personality is completely variable depending on the situation.

But the idea that what we look like is somehow irrelevant, not serious, or not important, to me, is disingenuous. We are visual creatures as humans, which is a great gift, not something that should be judged as superficial. Ultimately it is the INTEGRATION of the inner and outer that has always been my guiding light.

If we realize that our outer self is as unique as our inner self, then we have to understand that there are no "flaws." No "mistakes." No "accidents."

Furthermore, I put out to you that it's our very unique makeup that IS our beauty. Beauty is about being the ONE AND ONLY YOU! This means SELF-ACCEPTANCE is not only essential, it's our natural state of being.

We come to earth as little bundles of pure love! No judgments. No preconceptions. No prejudices. We just exist in a state of LOVE. A baby doesn't arrive here wishing it was someone else. It just IS itself.

All nature's creations live in the total legitimacy of what they are. A rose doesn't expend any energy wishing it was a lily. It spends its entire life simply blossoming in the way it was fashioned to be.

It's only humans, in our infinite "wisdom" that devolve into a *fear-based* sense of identity. The concepts of "being less than," "flaws," "mistakes," corrective techniques, etc. are all in direct opposition to the harmony nature has created for us to thrive in.

Yet these fear-based premises are what all the traditional beauty and style rules are based on. Women have been tortured since the beginning of time with the dictates that thrive on the horrible concept of beauty being false ideals that exist outside the self and the idea that your beauty can only be achieved by reaching for that standard. The techniques required to do this involve hiding, covering up, correcting, etc. These are all sadly (and ineffectively) fear-based methods. Their very existence requires you to be convinced in the first place that there is something you lack.

Following these dictates always results in low self-esteem. After all, if you aren't the "ideal," then your efforts, even at their best, are just a façade, a false presentation over the "real you" hidden underneath. This means, of course, you are left feeling less than. What a horrible (and false) effect!

Pretty awful to consider that all traditional beauty/style rules are based on making you feel insecure!

From the very beginning of my career, I rejected all these false constraints and began developing new techniques. Mustering up all my history and the expertise I acquired from my years as an artist, I set about creating a new and completely original approach.

Starting with the foundation of *Working in Harmony with Nature*. This radical approach revises all the old tenets that were based on shortcomings and replaces them with the magic, power, and joy contained in the idea that *There are no flaws, only unique characteristics*!

Having now withstood the test of time, I happily am inviting you to discover the magic, the power, and the absolute joy of LOVE-BASED BEAUTY.

YOU ARE A STAR—IT'S YOUR BIRTHRIGHT!

> *We are made of star stuff.*
> —CARL SAGAN

> *We are stardust brought to life.*
> —NEIL DEGRASSE TYSON

Billions of years ago, major stars exploded and scattered their mass across the galaxies, creating life here on Earth as we know it. Humans and stars are made up of the same four elements: hydrogen, oxygen, nitrogen, and carbon. This is a scientific fact long since proven and championed by astrophysicists.

So, when I say to you that YOU ARE THE STAR OF YOUR LIFE, I am not speaking metaphorically—it is literal. Your life is the chance to transform from the baby star that is your birthright into the blazing sun you have been given the breathtaking opportunity to become.

Each of us comes to this planet as an individual, the one and only YOU. You come with a purpose, which only YOU can fulfill by *telling your story*—in the way that you, and only you, can tell it.

BUT—you cannot tell your story in a vacuum. While you are indeed the STAR of your own story, you are far from a solo act. Your story is NOT just about how you experience yourself.

Everyone you come into contact with is a supporting character in your tale. *Your story cannot come to pass without their participation.* Furthermore, each one of them is simultaneously starring in their own personal story, of which YOU are a supporting character. One's story cannot fulfill itself alone. It requires the CONNECTION to others to take place.

Just as the heavens contain a multitude of stars all blazing concurrently, fueling life in the universe, we humans are always acting in tandem, weaving our lives into one fabulous tapestry that is constantly becoming the epic of our time on this planet.

This is the fabric of life. We are all creating together. We need each other's story to thrive. The world suffers when any one of us remains silent. All of our stories are incomplete, unless we invite each other to claim their parts.

The success and fulfillment of our stories depend on how we communicate them to each other.

This is where STYLE *comes into the picture.*

THE PATHWAY TO YOUR DREAMS

THE ASPIRATION OF STYLE

The Sibling and the Rival: Fashion and Trend

STYLE is often confused and conflated with Fashion and Trend. While there is a link between the three, they are each separate (but not equal!) animals.

Sibling FASHION, at its best, can mirror the times we live in. That's why we can instantly perceive a specific era from a photo or a film just by the clothing. The greatest designers of all time can turn fashion into art. Today, however, since conglomerates control all the labels, fashion is more business than art, with the creation of each collection playing second fiddle to the marketing of it.

Rival TREND is all about making the fast buck and keeping it coming. It thrives on social media convincing women of an unrelenting need to keep up with what's hot and has nothing to do with excellence of design or purpose. Constant turnover and planned obsolescence are its generators. *Today's trends are already yesterday's news!*

STYLE, on the other hand, has a much more overarching purpose that both FASHION and TREND lack. It's aspirational, combining not simply who you are today but who you yearn to be.

More than simply the way you dress, style incorporates your entire being—your IDENTITY, the integration of your inner and outer selves. It is the visual language with which you express everything you embody.

Your style, unlike fashion or trend, is timeless. Your style will (and must) certainly evolve, as we all change through life. But, because its foundation is based on your IDENTITY, rooted in your body and soul, it is not subject to the seasonal revamps of fashion or the unrelenting cycles of trend.

Instead, the understanding of your style allows you to borrow the parts of fashion *that serve your purpose,* so you can perform necessary updates. And if there comes a trend that is delightful to you, you will have the control of your style destiny to trip lightly through that minefield without being suckered into it!

STYLE IS YOUR SUPERPOWER

YOU ARE A MAGNET!

> *You contain a magnetic power within you that is more powerful than anything in this world.*
>
> —RHONDA BYRNE

To start, let's begin to understand what style actually is.

Style, at its core, is really COMMUNICATION— how you visually "tell your story." It's how you claim your purpose in life and how you tell it to the world. It's about your CONNECTION with others. It's the visual expression of your identity, and it must be able to evolve as you evolve.

It's not just about your "feeling." It always must include the outward connection to the world.

Style is NOT *"Look at me!"* That's the self-absorption of Instagram and social media, where everything is about gaining "likes" and chasing after trends. What passes for an influencer's style is often really just based on shock value and vanity. "Trend for trend's sake," rather than sharing what is one's actual intrinsic style.

Even simply walking down the street, you exist *not just by yourself.* The sidewalk is not private property! It's a communal space where we all share our experience. You are reaching out to the world and putting your energy out there. We *always* are interchanging energy (albeit mostly by default). When you understand the power of style and harness it, you automatically are sending waves of love out. STYLE IS SHARING YOUR LIGHT WITH THE WORLD!

YOUR STYLE IS ASPIRATIONAL— AND TIMELESS.

THE VITALS OF STYLE

YOUR THREE SELVES

Now, in case you're thinking I'm suggesting that your style is all about how others see you, let me divest you completely of that notion. Absolutely not!

Your style starts with YOU. It emanates entirely from your core IDENTITY. If we are going to talk about Love-Based Beauty, then the love must start with yourself.

The core of your style must emanate from: 1) Self Love. 2) Self-Acceptance. 3) Self-Celebration. These are the three seeds from which your style will flower. Without these three starting points, there is no possibility of AUTHENTICITY, which is essential to developing your style. *(Authenticity is always the one crucial component that separates Style from just a "Look.")*

I believe we are naturally predisposed to these, although, sadly, our histories tend to have made us bury them so deep we have mostly forgotten their existence.

We have to learn how to bring these up and out again, in order to start to build the process of developing your true style. However, that is just the beginning. For you to unleash the full power, you also need to embrace this fact:

TRUE STYLE IS INCLUSIVE.

Ultimately, however, how you feel in your skin, your taste, and your likes are just the beginning point. The idea "I wear whatever I want, and that's my style" is *incomplete and actually a false assumption.*

When it stops with the focus solely on you, *it's narcissistic* in nature. Certainly, people should have the freedom and the joy of loving what they wear, but keeping your entire focus inward keeps you wrapped up in yourself.

The simple action of including your surroundings and considering the IMPACT you can have on your fellow humans is going to take your style to the level you cannot imagine! INCLUSION *is what will lead to your* EMPOWERMENT.

STYLE IS ENERGY

Style, like everything else in life, is, at its essence, energy. When your focus is solely on yourself, your style is static. Your energy is dull, lifeless. It remains in place.

True style is cyclical. The energy starts with you, reaches out to others, and then returns tenfold. Just think of the magnitude you create when your style is about embracing others. Then the energy you create with it is electric!

When your style is rooted in your IDENTITY, you also are like a walking, talking magnet.

Love-Based Beauty combined with the power of FOCUS sends your dreams right out to those of like minds. You bring the people who are hungry for your story right to your doorstep. This cannot fail to materialize, because love begets love when your style is INCLUSIVE.

You also change the world in ways you cannot even realize. Whenever Susan and I are out and about, watching little girls (around the age of six) stop and give her a look of wonder and delight, I always tell Susan, "You just changed that little girl's life. That image of you is embedded in her brain." I'm reminded how powerful certain moments from childhood remain with us forever and of the influence ones from my life have had.

I want you to always be including *sharing the sidewalk* as your approach to your style. It will reap untold rewards in your life. Most important, you will discover how fulfilling it is to share your beauty with the world. That's the biggest gift of all—the change in your EXPERIENCE.

AUTHENTICITY IS THE CRUCIAL COMPONENT THAT SEPARATES STYLE FROM JUST A "LOOK."

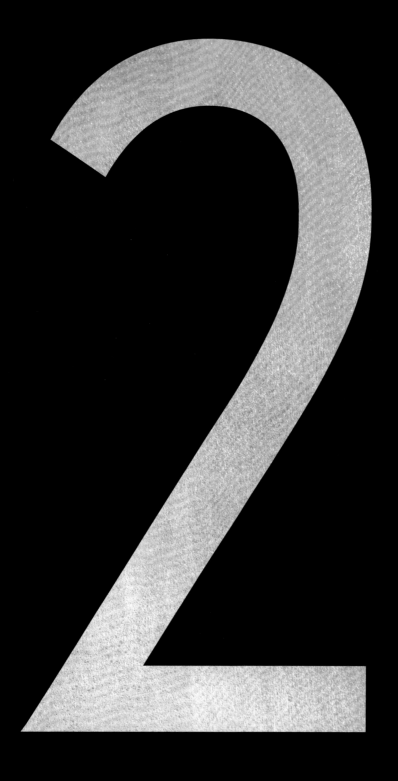

PART

2

THE NUTS
AND BOLTS
OF
STYLE

PREAMBLE: THE METAMORPHOSIS OF THE SYSTEM

A.K.A. THE JOURNEY OF YESTERDAY TO TODAY

> *To exist is to change, to change is to mature, to mature is to go on creating oneself endlessly.*
>
> —HENRI BERGSON

I've been privileged to have been doing this work for four decades. That's over forty years of *getting up every day and working to make this program better*. Not just in theory, but in practice. (I've not spent these years just writing or espousing about it in interviews!)

I'm actually in the field every day, working with new and old clients, consulting with them and guiding their transformations, a part of which involves being in the stores with them as we create their wardrobes. This means as the clothes are ever-changing, *I am in a constant state of updating*. It comes with the territory.

I also spend considerable time reading and researching, both to mine the treasure trove of the historical roots of style as well as harnessing new technology and societal changes in order to hone and elevate the process.

In short, as the world evolves, so must we all. So have I. So have my techniques. While style (and the principles that create it) is timeless, it must evolve as the world evolves. That is an essential part of the meaning of style. It is never set in stone. Your style cannot be static; therefore, your style, and this technique, must always be in process.

In 1987, my first book, *David Kibbe's Metamorphosis,* was released. I am both humbled and honored that in the years that have transpired, it has become such a beloved companion and source of inspiration to so many throughout the world. Each decade since has brought a new generation into the process as it's been rediscovered, and with the advent of social media, its outreach has expanded beyond what was even imaginable back at its inception.

TRY TO LEAVE BEHIND WHAT YOU THINK YOU KNOW!

THAT WAS THEN, THIS IS NOW!

However, as gratifying as this latest renaissance has been, it's time to realize that that was then, this is NOW. While the principles and underlying philosophy are certainly the same (and always will be), my methodology and worldview have both advanced exponentially.

There are so many things that have changed that couldn't have been imagined since the publication of the old book. In all these years, I've always been keeping things moving along to change as the world changed around me.

This means there are a number of things from my earlier book that have been wholly reimagined in this book—some updated elements, some revised elements, some entirely new techniques.

Technology alone has demanded a need for an approach to dressing that didn't exist until now. It has invented previously nonexistent fabrics today that require an entirely new way of clothing the body.

Thankfully, the world has also realized it must become more inclusive in its aspirations, in terms of both multicultural design and expanding the range of beauty standards.

While a major part of my work has always been based upon the ultimate inclusivity of the concept that beauty comes from individuality, with today's vision, we are able to be more adamant and provide more clarity in how to express this.

Social media has revolutionized the landscape while also being a double-edged sword. It's been a conduit to freedom while also providing a megaphone for balderdash.

On the one hand, the direct link with women it has given me has been the laboratory to create the new, game-changing techniques that make up this book. It's allowed those techniques to be tested in real time and proven to create fabulous results.

On the flip side, social media has also become an echo chamber of flat-out wrong information. It magnifies the myths, misdirects, misleads, and falsehoods. It also provides fertile ground for going down crazy rabbit holes.

CHANGE IS IN THE AIR!

"Don't be afraid, change is such a beautiful thing," said the butterfly.
—SABRINA NEWBY

So, let's view this as a brand-new chance to discover all the marvelous wonders nature has blessed you with. Be sure that you keep your focus on what's actually being presented here. Try to leave what you *"think you know"* behind. If you bring outside information into our journey, you will defeat the purpose.

All that's required for this to work for you is that you approach things with an *open mind,* an *open heart,* and a *willingness to change.* This is key.

I'm not saying you HAVE to change. I'm merely saying you must be WILLING to change. It is, of course, entirely up to you.

So, time for some getting-down-to-basics fun!

TECHNIQUE

THE GATEWAY TO YOUR FREEDOM

At thirteen, I was given a seminal life lesson in the critical part technique plays in realizing our potential. Without this, we might not actually be traveling this journey today!

I was already long considered a piano prodigy, winning awards, playing recitals, and such. At this time, I was awarded a scholarship to a prestigious music camp at a university with a storied piano division. Even though I was the youngest, I was chosen to play in the big recital and hand-picked for lessons with the head of the department. At his overview, he gave me the advice that changed my life.

"David, you have music oozing out of every pore. However, at this point, your fingers can't quite convey the depth of your talent." Then, gingerly, he told me I needed to change teachers to find one who could develop the proper technique that would set my talent free. (A music student's relationship to their teacher is always a tricky subject to broach!)

Well, I took his advice and found my new teacher, one of the greats, who taught me the technique that has fueled not only my music but all my life's accomplishments. (The very foundation of Love-Based Beauty has a direct link to what I learned via my beloved mentor.) *Talent and potential lie dormant without the conduit of technique to bring them forth!*

STYLE IS AN ACQUIRED SKILL

Style is not innate, it's learned. No one pops out of the womb with savoir faire! I know it may be hard to believe, but Fred Astaire didn't leap out of his cradle wearing a top hat and tails.

Our style is developed over time, as we discover all the things that make us tick and learn how to translate them into a visible form. It's not just our taste, what we like, or some inborn sensibility. These are mercurial (sometimes mythical) things, subject to whims, and they don't communicate our complete self.

When people base their idea of their style on what they are used to, they are actually crippled by limited vision. Style is NEVER what one is used to. It's always in the discovery of our POTENTIAL that we are ultimately transformed.

It's not about who we are but who we can become. What we bring into this world is like our raw material. It's what we learn to do with our natural riches that creates our style.

So, what we have to do is, first, *identify the two parts of ourselves* that are essential to our style: the inner and the outer. How you learn to FOCUS these and make them visible is the key. This is exactly what I designed this entire program of Love-Based Beauty to do: to capture all the elements of YOU and literally put them into your appearance. It's the process of TRANSFORMATION, step by step.

THE DO-IT-YOURSELF METHOD (DIY)

DIY VS. ANALYSIS

There are two (and only two) ways of making Love-Based Beauty work for you: 1) Doing it yourself: the DIY method. 2) Being professionally analyzed (correctly) by a certified consultant.

To be accurately analyzed, you need someone trained to look at you both with the complete knowledge of all the elements of my method as well as having learned to see you through a detached and educated eye. *This requires someone authorized and certified as a Kibbe consultant. It takes a very specifically taught skill to do this.*

There is no such thing as an analysis without this proper certified training. However well-meaning, without proper certification, anything else is only one person's faulty guess. As we will learn in just a bit, everyone sees through *our own subjective vision.* This way of looking at you (without the training) is going to be flawed, and send you down unending rabbit holes of misinformation.

Any one person or group attempting to *tell* you the elements that create your style should always be considered an attempt at an unskilled analysis. It will never be accurate. It's not possible.

The one method that does work, besides a professional consultation, is for you to uncover things yourself. You CAN do this, if you have the proper method.

This is the DIY approach, which is what this book is all about! (Don't confuse this with being a training manual for consultants. That's an entirely different process requiring a completely different set of skills that are not being presented here.)

THIS DIY METHOD IS A GUIDED JOURNEY OF PERSONAL DISCOVERY FOR YOU TO TRAVEL.

Each stage allows you to uncover the elements that lead to your style. It's a step-by-step approach that allows you to go at your own pace. I like to describe it as a JOURNEY OF JOY because it reveals a new vision of yourself that comes from your heart. You discover things in the way that you, and only you, can know about yourself. These discoveries are like continual gifts of delight!

The benefits of DIY are that you have the chance to integrate things along the way. It is a very organic approach where each step manifests and naturally rolls over to the next. *All you need to do is follow the instructions and allow the process to unfold.*

It's sort of like putting a jigsaw puzzle together piece by piece. By simply continuing the process, the picture begins to emerge until: Voilà! It's YOU in all your glory.

The other great gift I believe you get to receive is that the DIY approach is like a reawakening of things you knew somehow but have perhaps forgotten along the winding path of life. There are many "Aha!" moments along the way that become the basis of your transformed sense of self. These are things no one can tell you. You must (and will) EXPERIENCE them for yourself.

The journey of discovering your style is truly the process of undergoing a personal metamorphosis. We are all Nature's children, and she has given us each a built-in possibility of transforming into our most glorious self. It may seem a bit like a cliché to say we are budding butterflies, but that is honestly the truth. Each of us, in our own way, is designed to soar through life, sharing our special gifts with the world!

BEAUTY IS IN THE EYE OF THE BEHOLDER

A few years ago, my wife, Susan, and I went to support a friend's exhibition at a New York museum. A video portion showcased three adult sisters in individual clips sharing memories of the same afternoon on their father's boat.

The youngest sister rhapsodized on and on: "My father had this enormous yacht, so luxurious." The second sister dismissed it as, "He had this crummy little boat, barely able to fit us into." The third simply reported, "My father had a fishing boat."

We laughed so hard viewing this. It was a vivid illustration of the principle I often share with people online when they go on forever arguing about color definitions. Ask five people to name a color and you'll get five different answers.

Beauty truly is in the eye of the beholder. It's always about everyone's unique and different PERCEPTION.

When it comes to STYLE, OBJECTIVITY IS A HOAX!

As human beings, we all EXPERIENCE life. At our core being, we are visceral creatures. We are hardwired this way. We can't escape this fact. And we would not want to if we could. The beauty of humanity is how we emotionally relate to life and each other. The wonder of life is EXPERIENCED through our senses.

We *taste* that luscious gelato. We *rhapsodize* over a glorious cloud formation. We *bask* on a sun-drenched beach. We *inhale* the scent of fresh-baked bread. Furthermore, both our experiences and our descriptions of them are always personal, *unique to the person undergoing them*. This makes us all subjective creatures. As we will discover momentarily, it's our very subjectivity that is our ace in the hole!

There is no universal standard of experience, definition, or vision. There is no such thing as objectivity in terms of our perception. Objectivity is an intellectual concept that has no relevance to our style. *That is vital to understand in our journey.*

You cannot see yourself, or anyone else, objectively. It is impossible. We can, however, learn to work around that, but first *we must eliminate objectivity as a goal*. We have to dispel the myths about objectivity as a possibility when it comes to style.

THERE'S MORE TO YOU THAN MEETS THE EYE

"MIRROR, MIRROR ON THE WALL"

An update/rework of *Snow White*'s evil queen–and-mirror confab:

You: "Mirror, mirror on the wall, who's the fairest of them all?"

Mirror (in your mother's voice): "Well, darling, you do have that 'distinctive' nose, and then your hips— well, you're such a dear little 'pear.' . . . Now, your cousin Alice [sigh], she has those perfect features. But, sweetheart, you have a lovely smile."

None of us see ourselves, or others, in an impartial way. *We see through the lens of our history.* What you see in the mirror is a collection of distortions. (It's the same in video and photos.) These so-called mirrors merely present you a tampered-with picture. It's not YOU.

First, what a mirror shows you is in reverse—and that is just the initial distortion. You cannot ever receive an accurate reflection of what you look like.

Next, what a mirror is offering up to you is just an

image that's being filtered through every bit of your life's experience.

It's reflecting all the things about you that are not "ideal"; what you wish you were, or maybe what your mother wished you were! Every flaw you've been brainwashed into believing you exhibit is being falsely offered up as the "real" you.

Photos are just as misleading. *The camera tricks the eye.* I have spent years on both sides of the camera, in all media, and can attest to how difficult it is to capture what a subject actually looks like.

Years ago, the top headshot photographer for actors in New York had printed on his business cards "Photos twice as real as reality." The work he put into getting shots that actually looked like the actor was unbelievable.

(The great news here is that those photos you cringe at—that's not at all what you look like!)

You are never going to be able to see either yourself or anyone else without the distortion of your subjective vision. Likewise, the way everyone else sees you is also always skewed. They are ALWAYS viewing you through their own biased perception.

NO QUIZZES, NO TYPING!

This imprecise vision is the reason quizzes and so-called "typing" are guaranteed to set you on a wild-goose chase! Round and round you will go, getting false answers and an overabundance of contradictory pronouncements.

"Typing" is a faulty premise to begin with. That's shorthand for stereotyping, which is the very opposite of everything that Love-Based Beauty was created to achieve. You are an individual, NOT a "type." It's a wrongheaded notion seen through flawed perceptions. As I previously stated, analysis can only correctly be done by someone who is correctly trained. A "typing," by either an untrained person or a group, is only a subjective guess *based on incomplete information.*

As for quizzes, the very premise of a quiz is to test what you already know. It's NOT to provide you with answers to things. Think about your school days.

You studied information, then took a test to see what you'd retained from what you studied.

You have to know the correct answers BEFORE you take a quiz. You cannot receive an accurate result from taking a test if you don't already know the correct answers to each question.

So let's put the old and unworkable ideas of quizzes and typing to bed. They don't work. They can't work. They are dead to you and me and hereby banished to permanent detention, where all old-style rules go to contemplate their misdeeds!

In their place, I want to introduce you to a whole new approach to discovering and developing your style. One that is rooted in the AUTHENTICITY of your soul and allows the full EMPOWERMENT of your purpose. We are going to learn to replace faulty vision with AUTHENTIC EXPERIENCE.

REPLACE FAULTY VISION WITH AUTHENTIC EXPERIENCE.

THE *EXPERIENCE* OF YOU

EMBRACING YOUR SUBJECTIVITY

So, as we realize the concept of objectivity is non-existent, how do we discover what we need to learn about ourselves in order to reach our style goals?

I'm going to lead you through an altogether different method that not only accepts your subjectivity as your natural state of being but also considers it an advantage that can be incorporated into achieving your goal. It is based on literally EMBRACING your subjectivity as the basis of achieving your ultimate transformation.

What I'm going to give you is a *brand-new way to define yourself*. One that doesn't require the hoax of an objective vision. *What we are going to do is learn to replace what you* think you see *with how you* EXPERIENCE *yourself!*

Now, first, let's define what I mean by EXPERIENCE. It's not feeling, but it is visceral. It's not intellectual, but it does involve learning. It's not about how others see you, but it does include connecting with others.

It happens via a series of games that are played, which have a built-in gain. You will find you have CHANGED just by playing each game the way it's laid out. Each one will reveal the things about you that will become the building blocks that develop your style. As you simply play the games, you will be creating the MASTERPIECE that is YOU!

In the end, style cannot be assigned or given. Even with a first-rate professional analysis, your style is *developed*. It always involves an integration of the WHOLE AUTHENTIC SELF. That's why my DIY technique achieves such amazing results. It is the actual step-by-step process that unfolds with everything simply *built-in*. When you move through it via your EXPERIENCE, it cannot help but be authentic to you. Furthermore, the transformation involved will all occur by design.

This is going to be a transformative process based on three things: 1) uncovering and defining the false assumptions you have integrated that have held you back; 2) learning a new way to experience your authentic self and see things through *loving eyes;* 3) bringing your dreams to life as you discover the true superpower of your style.

So, first, let's learn a bit more about the nature of our subjectivity and how we can harness it.

THE THREE STAGES OF SUBJECTIVITY

1. **EMBRACING SUBJECTIVITY AS OUR NATURAL STATE OF BEING.** The starting point. We accept we are always subjective.

2. **LEARNING THE STATE OF *INTELLIGENT SUBJECTIVITY*.** This is where we learn techniques that allow us to use our subjectivity to move us forward.

3. **ARRIVING AT THE STATE OF *ENLIGHTENED SUBJECTIVITY*.** These are the "AHA!" moments when it all comes together. You experience the empowerment of your style as it is realized. It is where the inner and outer become aligned.

The Three Stages of Subjectivity are the *why* behind the creation of what's to come. How I've utilized them to move you forward is the territory we are now entering, the land where we can discover the more accurate versions of what is to become part and parcel of your style: *your Season, your Image Identity, and all the other tangible pieces that go into creating it.*

This is my reimagined way we can ensure all these are legitimately yours!

MOVING FROM THE *WHY* INTO THE *HOW*

So far, we've been concentrating on the why and what of our journey, understanding the need for this new model of beauty. As we move forward into the *how,* it's essential that we remember all we've learned so far that is the basis and the reasoning for this new approach. We must be diligent to never slip back into old ideas or rules we are used to. A revolutionary concept of Love-Based Beauty requires brand-new tools!

NEW TOOLS
Working in Harmony with Nature

With our guiding light being *Working in Harmony with Nature,* I've designed our new tools with three purposes: to ENHANCE, CLARIFY, and FOCUS. This is now our strategy for what follows. 1) Enhance your natural beauty, 2) Clarify it with the new technique, 3) resulting in the Focus that allows it to be visually communicated to the world.

Remember when earlier I mentioned we need to capture both your inner and outer selves to create your style? While ultimately it is the integration of both, since they are innately different in their makeup, we need two different methods to translate them.

Your inner self is *ephemeral.* Volatile and ever-changing, it is an abstract energy that can't be expressed directly or captured via a confined structure. *We focus it through a situational approach,* which I will be guiding you through.

Since your outer self is *tangible* and more fixed, we'll start there.

First, let's IDENTIFY yourself. Start by realizing you are a Masterpiece! Now think of yourself as both a PAINTING and a SCULPTURE—color and form. (In other words, your coloring is your painting, and your form is your sculpture.)

So basically, we simply employ harmonious colors to your painting and complementary outlines to your form. We call your painting your SEASON and your sculpture your IMAGE IDENTITY.

Now, here's where we need a new method to discover both for you, as well as awaken you to all the fabulous potential you have and bring your dreams to life. Here are my new tools that will take you to the heights where your style can emerge in all its glory! So, throw off the yoke of the old and get ready to embrace the unlimited freedom of the new.

This is INTELLIGENT SUBJECTIVITY at work!

YOU ARE A PAINTING AND A SCULPTURE!

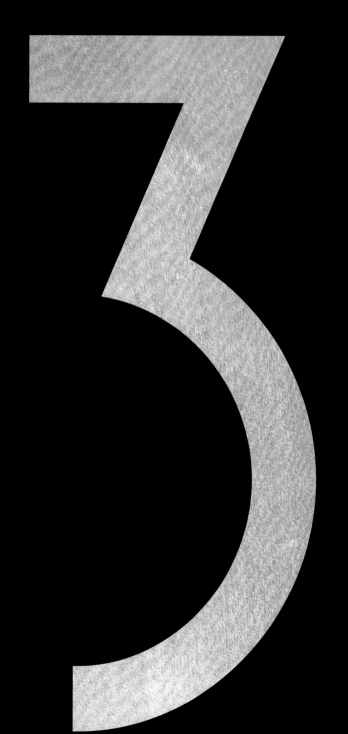

PART

3

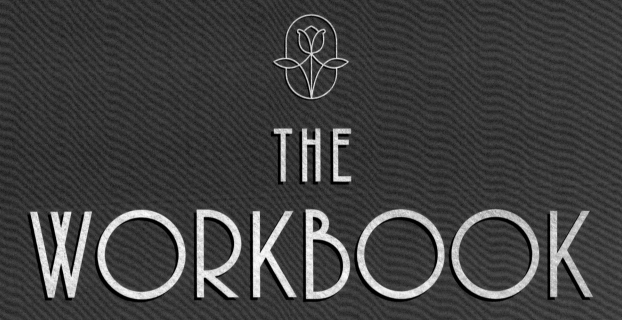

THE
WORKBOOK

PRELUDE: THE GAMES

"PLAYING" YOUR WAY TO STYLE

> The creation of something new is not accomplished by the intellect but by the play instinct.
>
> —CARL JUNG

What you need now is a new approach to HOW you see yourself. Since the old-style quizzes and "type me" determinations can never be accurate (*objectivity is a hoax*), we have to find a new mirror of yourself that is based on something real, something that is steadfast and cannot be challenged. *You need to find a new way to view yourself that reveals what is authentically you.*

The GAMES are that way!

AUTHENTICITY IS YOUR NEW MIRROR

A surefire way of ensuring authenticity is to connect it to how you EXPERIENCE something. Your personal experience is always authentic. It CAN'T be anything else. It's YOUR experience.

And the best way to create an authentic experience for yourself is to simply undergo a SITUATION, a specific circumstance you find yourself in. An event is usually involved, but it always includes an environment surrounding you as well as anything that you would have natural reactions to. The way you experience a situation *always* will reveal truths about yourself that are absolutely authentic. (And more often than not, they are also hidden.)

So I created this series of games for you to play with the one purpose simply being *to obtain the experience of playing them*. All you have to do is play the game as it's laid out, and you've achieved its purpose!

Each one is situational, designed with a built-in goal that occurs automatically. *You don't "work for it" or try for a certain result.*

Your only task is to follow instructions. Don't add, subtract, skip over, or improvise. You do need to actually DO them. You can't *think* them through to receive the result.

Remember, there is one goal: your EXPERIENCE. That's the only thing that counts here. The gain happens on its own.

Some games will challenge your preconceptions. Some will bring up prejudices that are limiting your possibilities. Some will give you awesome new insights. Some will open up magical new worlds of possibilities. Some will absolutely blow your mind! They are all transformational and each one moves you forward, rolling into the next. In the end, it is the sum total that will have completely expanded and changed the way you see yourself (and, quite possibly, the world around you).

What they all will do is give you the AUTHENTIC information about yourself that will take you right up to the point of discovering your SEASON and your IMAGE IDENTITY in ways you simply could never have gotten to before. The games will also open the ultimate ways they can be expressed, ways that will have heretofore been unimagined!

Since these are wholly new methods, I'm sure

you will have many feelings coming up along the way. *Don't worry, there is room for all of them.* It's all in the mix, by design. There is no *right or wrong* and absolutely no judgment. This is all simply part of your personal journey.

NOW VERY IMPORTANT: PLEASE HAVE FUN. PLAY THE GAMES. This is the reason for their design. Don't view them as homework.

Here we go! Off to the races!

YOUR PREGAME WARM-UP

TUNING UP YOUR INSTRUMENT

1. **GO TO ZERO**

2. **CONJURE UP YOUR MOMENT OF AWE**

3. **DO SUSAN'S BREATH OF LIFE**

Just like a singer does vocal warm-ups before a performance or rehearsal, or a jogger does stretches before a run, you are going to want to do a little warming up before you start to play each game. In our endeavors, this means you need to start by getting centered in your love-based core. *You need a relaxed, open channel for all the magic to pour through!*

Once you define these warm-ups, they will only take you a few moments. But these few moments will turbocharge your success! *It's always starting in the right frame of mind and right state of body that is the key to capturing the power of these games.* Forgo them and you will end up wasting a lot of time going in wrong directions. The time you will squander meandering and going down endless rabbit holes can be totally eradicated by just taking a few moments to start with these gentle pregame warm-ups.

Note: Let's preface this by giving credit where credit is due: These are all adapted from the technique Susan created at her revolutionary acting school. She originated all of these marvelous techniques and is responsible for the fantastic results each gives.

GROUND ZERO

START WHERE YOU ARE TO GO FAR

This is called *going to zero*. Sit back in a chair. Relax. Shut your eyes and let everything go. Let your mind go blank. Let your body go slack. Breathe very gently and just feel yourself at one with your surroundings. Gently nudge away any thoughts that come up. Release all pressure to achieve anything. *Revel in the passive pleasure of emptiness, of total neutrality.* This is ALWAYS YOUR STARTING POINT. We will be referring to this from now on by saying "GO TO ZERO."

YOUR MOMENT OF AWE

A GLIMPSE OF YOUR BLISS

This is simply to define a visual picture of an image from your life that fills you with AWE. It can be a person, a place, an object, even a food! It is simply one visual that, as you see it, inspires that deep sense of unworldly bliss. But it's the FEELING in your BODY the image elicits that we are looking to identify.

Now, BE SPECIFIC, not general or generic. Start by identifying the situation the image occurred in, then isolate the ONE specific picture from that situation.

Here's an example from my life. My situation: I love the tropics. I have one place Susan and I have returned to several times. On our balcony, the view of the sea and the clouds hanging so low I'm sure I can reach out and grab them immediately transports me. My awe image: those clouds.

It doesn't hurt to have a backup, just because sometimes you get more juice from changing it up. Here's my backup (which is another that never fails to get me *right there*!). The Situation: My wedding day, which was in our apartment. The image: The appearance of Susan, looking like a glamorous angel resplendent in white and shimmering silver.

Again, it can be anything. I have a friend who gets weak in the knees at the very mention of a hot fudge sundae! I'm sure her number one awe image would be drawn from her vast experience of sundae hunting!

Here's an optional addition to this for music lovers. Hearing the opening of a piece you love can be a very powerful secondary moment of awe. For me, when I hear the first strains of Pachelbel's Canon in D, I am instantly enraptured. I have a friend who can't stop herself from getting up and dancing as soon as she hears the first bars of Aretha's "Respect." Music can be a powerful bliss jolter! When it comes to conjuring up your awe moment, it never hurts to have more than one iron in your fire!

Just remember, *it's how your body reacts to the image that is the key to this warm-up.* You've got to pick an image that elicits this feeling. You'll have these images in your back pocket to use as needed. We will be calling this PULLING UP YOUR AWE.

SUSAN'S BREATH OF LIFE

YOUR CIRCLE OF LOVE

This is a variation of Susan's version of a popular deep-breathing exercise. She starts every joint session we do with a more extended version of this vital warm-up. It gets all of us aligned in the same energy before we begin. *Your life force is instantly activated by connecting to your breath. To soar, you always must start in your center, and as human beings, that's our heart.*

Sit in a chair with both feet planted on the ground, and lean back with your eyes shut and relax. Gently start breathing with a slow, deep inhalation through the nose. Hold a second at the height of the inhale, then release on a slow, deep exhalation through the mouth. As you repeat, inhale on the count of three, hold for two, exhale on a count of five. As you get comfortable, breathe in the word "YES!" (all the yeses of your possibilities). Then, as you exhale, send your "Yes!"es out into the world. (When you do this, expect them to come back to you tenfold.) Do this a couple of times. Then repeat the inhale, saying (in your head), "I CHOOSE LOVE"; hold; then keep that state of "I CHOOSE LOVE" as you gently exhale and sit for a moment in your center. You are now ready to begin! We will refer to this as DOING SUSAN'S BREATH.

Take a moment and practice these three tune-ups until you get them under your belt. Take your time until you feel comfortable with each. They are very pleasurable, so don't stress over any one. Go gently. When you actually use them before playing each game, you will only need to touch base with them to get you starting in the right place. These will center you. It will only take a couple of minutes to do these warm-ups at the start of every exercise.

A FRIENDLY WORD OF ADVICE AS WE BEGIN: Each game is very specifically designed down to the last detail. If you want to get the benefit from them, then please follow them exactly as they are laid out. There is a reason for everything that is included. There is also a reason for anything that is NOT included. Read the instructions carefully. And again, have FUN!

WE ARE PLAYMATES!

MY THREE LOVES

RESET OF YOUR VISION: *LOVING EYES*

Stand in front of a full-length mirror dressed in either a leotard, a bathing suit, or something similarly revealing. No makeup.

**CLOSE YOUR EYES AND
DO YOUR THREE WARM-UPS.**

1. **Go to zero.**

2. **Pull up your awe.**

3. **Do Susan's Breath.**

Now slowly open your eyes, and look at yourself through tender eyes. If any critical thoughts come up, gently push them aside. Tell yourself you can always come back to those thoughts, but for now, you want to find other, kinder ones. Find three things about your physical self that you love. They can be large things (such as "I love my legs") or small (such as "I love my right thumb").

When you identify each, spend a moment sending that part of your body caring energy. (An easy way is to simply caress that part while saying, "I love my nose," etc.) Then move on to the next part until you have finished all three. Do only three. No more. No less.

Then **WRITE THEM DOWN ON A SINGLE PIECE OF PAPER.** Put this in your purse or pocket, and carry it with you. It's important that you keep the list with you. Even though it is a tucked-away note, you will be aware you are carrying it with you. Every day, pull the note out and look at it once. This will help you remember how you felt when you gave support to that part of yourself in the mirror. Be consistent with this daily for three weeks. Then repeat this exercise in front of the mirror and notice any changes in your experience.

NOTE: It is **VITAL** that you write this down on paper. We will be using this later when we get to the shopping section. There will be an upcoming **THREE LOVES IN THE DRESSING ROOM!**

HANDY TIP: In a pinch, if you are flailing with this at any time, such as finding negative or critical thoughts coming up, take a deep breath, close your eyes, and repeat "I choose love" for a couple of moments. This will help recenter you in the *loving-eyes place* where you want to approach yourself. A hint: If you find yourself rolling your eyes at this, thinking it's just too corny, well, you're right, it is! However, *it is also unfailingly effective!* If you can't begin to learn to see yourself through loving eyes, nothing else we are going to do will have any lasting or genuine effect. *If you don't start with self-love, there is no chance for achieving authentic style.*

Style starts with YOU. Not an influencer. Not a celebrity. And it's not found "out there" somewhere. Before you can express it, you have to love the *subject*!

We are always our own worst critics. There has not been much of a lack in this area, historically.

How about now we work to become our own best friends? You were born loving yourself, unconditionally. Let's take some baby steps back in that direction!

It's a new day. From here on out, let's make a rock-solid commitment to see yourself with KINDER EYES.

MY THREE LOVES ARE

_____

_____

_____

_____

_____

_____

_____

_____

_____

_____

SEE YOURSELF WITH KINDER EYES!

LET'S GO TO THE MOVIES!

RAISING THE BAR

This game is just pure delight. I want you to simply sit back and revel in some great classic movies, from an era where style was a critical component to the very existence of the film. Where it wasn't so much about the re-creation of so-called reality as it was about transporting us to a world of big dreams and boundless imagination. Hollywood as America's dream factory.

There is a veritable gold mine of wealth for us in these films, but all I want you to do as you view them is just let them float over you. Just enjoy the experience. Don't try to decipher. And especially, DON'T try to *look at the costumes with the attitude of whether or not you think you would wear any of these things today.* That's not the purpose here at all.

Now, before we go forward, let me say I know that there are also many wonderful and worthwhile films today. There are also some fantastic designers who are great artists. The difference back then was in the studio system that created the films, the way they were created, and the reason for them. Today is different. Not less, just different. And what we are looking for in this game is dependent upon those differences.

Later on we will go into the impact of Old Hollywood on timeless style. There's a lot to be gained from the principles that were employed by those studios. There's also a lot lacking, sometimes shamefully so, from that era. When we get to that point, we will delve into both, as they are both critically necessary to understand in the development of your ultimate style. What's good, what's not good, and everything in between!

This game is not about those things, however. What I'm asking is that you just inhale the glorious artistry those genius designers employed in creating these spectacles. There is vision in them that we want to recapture and redeploy in our own journeys.

This game is actually about RAISING THE BAR. Remembering things that have been forgotten. And letting our dreams be as huge and joyous as our imagination allows.

Today, for lots of reasons, some of which are reasonable, some just sloppy, we have forgotten what is possible. Most of the time, we simply settle for what we know. I want to reintroduce you to what we can create when we allow ourselves to DREAM BIG.

We have let too many of our dreams deflate to miniature versions today. These films take us to heights we want to rescale—not in an imitative way, but rather, in an inspirational way. We can use these old films to nudge us to find new ways to bring grand dreams and unlimited possibilities to today's world. This game can move us to UP OUR GAME and RAISE OUR BAR!

The films to watch begin in the late 1930s, occur mainly in the forties and fifties, and end no later than the early to mid-sixties. (Of course, there are many other films with fabulous design; this is just a list that is specifically targeted for upcoming references along our journey.)

THE LIST

GIGI
Note the sumptuous overall use of color and design, and how characters were developed through style. (Also, any other Technicolor film directed by Vincente Minnelli will be valuable in showing the mastery of how unlimited vision is brought to life.)

FUNNY FACE
You have a trio of grand examples of specificity in Audrey Hepburn, Fred Astaire, and Kay Thompson. "Think Pink," Audrey's transformation, Fred's socks!

AN AFFAIR TO REMEMBER
Observe Deborah Kerr for exquisite examples of the clarity of ensemble/head-to-toe design, and of course Cary Grant for everything!

CARMEN JONES
Starring Dorothy Dandridge, for an abundance of dresses that are all very wearable to this very day. Daytime, but all with a glamorous touch.

THE WOMEN
For excellent character delineation. And the fashion show is zany but definitely a great example of the connection of "Situation to Outfit." This film is often way over the top, but it's fun and has wonderful examples of a great designer at his zenith. Make sure to view the original version starring Norma Shearer and Joan Crawford.

BORN YESTERDAY
A great example of showing many different facets of one person as Judy Holliday's multiple looks evolve.

STORMY WEATHER
and any other film with Lena Horne. (Mostly for gowns, as she is usually cast as a performer, but also for the design elements of the ensembles.)

PEYTON PLACE
Lana Turner version. Excellent example of 1950s "regular people" style. These designs are very much in the wearable-clothes category of that decade. Note the attention to detail, especially in the accessories. The clothes are all the same silhouette, very structured yet elegant. Also notice the great attention to the details of the hair and makeup design, which are timeless yet specific.

ADAM'S RIB
(Or any other Hepburn/Tracy films from the 1940s or '50s). Most American designers have a direct link to Katharine Hepburn.

Some designers worth exploring who personify the qualities we can learn from and use today: Edith Head, Adrian, Helen Rose, Irene Sharaff. They are all masters of character delineation, exquisite artistry, and absolute commitment to detail.

After viewing each film or clip, take a few moments to do your warm-ups as they will help put you in the perfect frame of mind to absorb the bounty that will be lavishing itself upon you! 1) Go to zero. 2) Pull up your awe. 3) Do Susan's Breath.

Then jot down anything that stands out to you in terms of the style components you just discovered. Especially note anything that was a new idea, a new sight. Note what brought you JOY. Think about what images you will carry with you as you recall the film.

This is how the gift from Raising the Bar will actually manifest as you progress. Take some time with this and really contemplate. *It will be a great resource when we get to the shopping portion and our ultimate creation of actual outfits with today's clothes.*

NOTE: Most of these films are available online for free. If you can't find them, you can easily find clips. But it's definitely far more valuable to watch the entire films. You can take your time with this game. Do try to watch at least two films and as many clips as you can before moving on. It will definitely open up your vision of what can be. ENJOY! (Popcorn, anyone?)

STANDOUTS FROM VIEWING

_____

_____

_____

_____

_____

_____

_____

_____

_____

_____

_____

_____

_____

_____

THE CARROT AND YOUR CAKE

DREAM IT TODAY, LIVE IT TOMORROW

What most people consider "reality" is just whatever they are used to. Yet, what we have accepted as "today's reality" didn't just happen by accident. Our experiences today weren't simply foisted upon us from some celestial dictatorship!

We are constantly fashioning our lives by our thoughts, images, and feelings, and **by our desires**. (And similarly, our style needs to be rooted in our desires to be truly ours.)

We created today's reality with the dreams we conjured up yesterday. (Now, more often than not we are continually doing this unconsciously, by default.)

If we created today with yesterday's thoughts, then RIGHT NOW, we are creating tomorrow. So, instead of simply accepting the status quo, how about we use our *elevated thought* to fuel our tomorrow?

Time to call on our DREAMS. Time to decide whether we want to be dream spinners or acquiescent vassals!

The power of our dreams is infinite. *They are only limited by the specificity of our desires.* Desire is the fuel. Our dreams are the tool. **Our dreams are images fueled by our desires.** That is why they are so

potent. *The surest link for developing our style is to hook into our dreams.*

Our dreams are our "carrots." We don't need them to be literal. Just like the farmer lured the proverbial donkey to the field with the promise of the luscious, glorious carrot, our dreams lead us, by our desires, to magical results that are beyond what we can predict.

Now, we want to remember that we've already defined style as always being personal to us, as well as aspirational. We never want to settle for anything less than *what can be*.

So, with that in mind, we are going to look back to what we gained from the last game (Let's Go to the Movies!) and use it as a springboard to this one.

I want you to use images that jazzed you from those movies (THE CARROT) to create new, inspired ideas for your life (YOUR CAKE).

I want you to learn to use your dreams and your desires to create your life. Not to simply settle for what you may be used to. *To reach to the stars for your reality!*

Here's the game:

THE CARROT:

Pick two images of stars in specific situations in films from the last game that thrill you, one daytime and one fancy.

YOUR CAKE:

Now, inspired by those specific star outfits/situations, create two outfits for specific situations for yourself.
(Create these outfits from sources anywhere online.)

Record your outfits on a scrapbook-type website (such as Pinterest) so you can see them. The only criterion is that you pick images that make you weak in the knees!

For example:

For your daytime star: You pick Lana Turner in the lilac tailored suit during her courtroom appearance in the film *Peyton Place*.

For your inspired daytime outfit: You pick a three-piece coordinated separate outfit from Zara (or any similar-price-point shop), a jacket/slacks/top outfit. In hot pink. (Keep this close to your budgetary range.)

For your fancy star: You pick Lena Horne in the showstopping asymmetrical one-shoulder white silk jersey gown with the leaf motif worn in one of her nightclub scenes in the film *Stormy Weather*.

For your inspired fancy outfit: You find a short, one-shoulder white silk dress that you could see yourself wearing to a cocktail party. (This could be a bit of a budget splurge!)

How you link your chosen *star outfit* to your personal one is up to you. It doesn't have to be as literal as my examples. Just make sure you have a real connection from the former to the latter. It's also important that you are specific to the situation in your life. That must not be general or vague.

Now, before we are finished, we have one more task. First, let's do the warm-up so we are coming from the best place to harvest this game.

1) Go to zero. 2) Pull up your awe. 3) Do Susan's Breath.

Now, from this centered and open place, identify, briefly, three different reasons that you chose your specific images and the links to your outfits. Then pare each of the three down to one word. (So you will end up with three different words.)

For instance, using the illustrations I gave above, the reason for the inspired daytime outfit could be: "*I chose Lana's suit because the color choice (lilac), combined with the tailoring, made a simple suit chic and elegant. It led me to find the hot-pink three-piece suit I got from Zara.*" The one-word distillation would be **COLOR**.

The reason for the inspired fancy outfit could be: "*I chose Lena's gown because the asymmetry of the shoulder makes me swoon. That's what made the one-shoulder design of my slinky cocktail dress sing to me.*" The one-word distillation would be **ASYMMETRY**.

The more specifically we identify the desires that make your heart sing, the more focused your style will become. We are distilling and harnessing your power! This is an important piece of your puzzle: using the **CARROT** of your desires and dreams to bake your **CAKE** (your style).

This game should be a total blast. It has no boundaries other than connecting the heart of your dreams to the actual reality of your life! **SHEER BLISS!**

Below, for "Your Carrot," record the name of the movie and the star that feature your inspirational outfit, and the one word that describes what captured your imagination. For "Your Cake," briefly describe the daytime outfit you created that was inspired by your movie and star, and include the one word you've used to connect it to your inspiration.

YOUR CARROT:
MY DAYTIME STAR
_____

_____

_____

_____

_____

YOUR CARROT:
MY FANCY STAR
_____

_____

_____

_____

_____

YOUR CAKE:
MY INSPIRED DAYTIME OUTFIT
_____

_____

_____

_____

_____

YOUR CAKE:
MY INSPIRED FANCY OUTFIT
_____

_____

_____

_____

_____

POTLUCK

PREJUDICES AND PRECONCEPTIONS WE BRING TO THE TABLE A.K.A. WE "SEE" WHAT WE LOOK FOR!

Two photographers taking a photo of the exact same image will each capture something entirely different. Why is that? *Because each one registers the very same object with a completely different vision.* Every human being sees everything through their own **SUBJECTIVE LENS.**

There is no universal way of seeing a person (whether it be yourself or anyone else). Five people will give you five completely different versions of what the same person looks like. Furthermore, each of the five will be *certain* their vision is correct! (In reality, none of them are!)

These differences, along with the "certainties," have nothing to do with what is actually there. They occur because *everyone brings their own particular prejudices and preconceptions to the table.* These are mostly unconscious, but they absolutely color our vision in every way, shape, and form.

In other words: WE "SEE" WHAT WE LOOK FOR!

The biggest handicap, as well as the reason for most of the mistakes people make in terms of identifying themselves physically, is the limited and prejudiced vision they start with.

So, the most important thing you can do **BEFORE** you even attempt to identify your physical self is to learn the prejudices and preconceptions you bring to the table that inform how you see yourself, both negative and positive.

In the last game, by connecting the images from the movies that thrilled you to the actual creation of outfits for yourself, you identified and then demonstrated the effect of positive preconceptions. This is exactly the way you will ultimately connect your inner essence and desires to your outer style. We will get to that later when we play our fantastical dream games!

Before that, however, it's vital for you to identify and understand how the negative prejudices and preconceptions limit your vision and actually are keeping you from realizing your true self!

So, here's what I want you to do: I am going to give you a list of words in two categories: **physical** and **descriptive**. I want you to discover whether you have a positive or negative reaction to each word and then pick the ones you have the most intense reaction to.

So here goes:

First, let's do your warm-up so your channel is open and you get the clearest results. 1) Go to zero. 2) Pull up your awe. 3) Do Susan's Breath.

Now that you're relaxed, look at these words and put them in two separate columns according to your reaction: POSITIVE (P) and NEGATIVE (N).

DESCRIPTIVE WORDS

Cute	Adorable
Powerful	Glamorous
Boyish	Girlish
Sexy	Strong
Understated	Soft
Sweet	Femme Fatale
Athletic	Diva
Brassy	Delicate
Innocent	Flamboyant
Trendy	Youthful

PHYSICAL WORDS

Shoulders	Petite
Hips	Broad
Thighs	Curvy
Bust	Short
Muscular	Sharp
Angular	Big
Thin	Small
Wide	Thick
Flesh	Waist
Curve	Long

Now that you've categorized these into 2 columns, Positive (P) and Negative (N), take another deep breath, take a moment, and locate the feeling each word elicits in your body. I want you to identify your visceral reactions to these words you've starred. Then go down each list and pick the four Ps and the four Ns that you have the most intense reaction to and star (*) these. That will be eight words in all.

What we have done now is identify your most deeply embedded preconceptions and prejudices, which will infuse your answers in the next section of games: the ones that determine your PERSONAL LINE, YIN/YANG, and IMAGE IDENTITY.

This game is IMPERATIVE for all else that follows. Without the benefit of it, you will never be able to overcome the handicaps that keep you from being able to accurately identify your physical qualities.

That being said, do play this game with a sense of excitement. This is going to be an eye-opener that will allow the magic of the unexpected and totally unforeseen to happen. Things beyond what you can imagine!

RECORD YOUR REACTIONS HERE (Note: There is no judgment here; the goal is only to recognize your instant reactions):

DESCRIPTIVE WORDS

POSITIVE REACTIONS (P)

_____

_____

_____

NEGATIVE REACTIONS (N)

_____

_____

_____

PHYSICAL WORDS

_____

_____

_____

_____

_____

_____

DING-DONG, RECESS!
(HIT THE PLAYGROUND)

TIME FOR A LITTLE BREATHER AND A RECAP (SO FAR, SO GREAT!)

I realize I'm asking a lot of you, my friends. Basically, to change everything you've ever learned and forget everything you thought you knew! Whew! How could I do this to you? Well, it's just that all I really want for you is the world!

So let's stop for a moment and take a breather to review all the amazing places we've already traveled to. And also let me give you super kudos for trusting me with your style journey so far.

First, we've discovered the NEW VISION that is LOVE-BASED BEAUTY. That alone is a game-changer. We've learned beauty comes from your individuality, and style is your way of expressing your unique purpose and place on our planet. (STYLE IS YOUR SUPERPOWER.)

It started with you (*We are STARDUST brought to life. . . .*), but it also reached out to include others. You saw it's primarily about communication and energy. (*Style is* INCLUSIVE; *You are a* MAGNET.)

We've realized TECHNIQUE is critical (style is an ACQUIRED SKILL). Since we became aware that it's impossible for us to be objective (Objectivity is a Hoax), we're learning a new approach that embraces our subjectivity as our greatest asset (Three Stages of Subjectivity). We've begun a method that doesn't rely on faulty vision but replaces that with an authentic way of discovering ourselves (the DIY approach, leading to a total EXPERIENCE of body and soul).

We've started to play the GAMES (DIY), which are uncovering, one by one, the pieces of our ultimate goal: the INTEGRATION OF INNER AND OUTER SELF that creates our STYLE.

First, we started off by warming up our channel to start each game with an open heart (pregame warm-up).

Then, to begin with, we laid the cornerstone of Love-Based Beauty: seeing ourselves through loving eyes (Three Loves). This is the foundation we build our house of style upon: *the bottomless well of self-acceptance.*

Then we gained aspiration from traveling back in time to the actual star-making factories (Let's Go to the Movies!). We identified new possibilities that thrilled us and *raised our bar* by rediscovering examples of great artistry that don't exist today.

Next, we learned how to take from the best of the past and bring it into today's world, updating, not replacing. We also practiced creating from JOY through choosing images that thrilled you (the Carrot and Your Cake).

Finally, we see that we limit ourselves and will continue to do so if we don't uncover and identify our prejudices and preconceptions. That these keep us from freedom and authenticity. Our biggest roadblock to unleashing our authentic style is what we "bring to the table" (Potluck).

So, while we have new ground to cover, especially as we get down to the basics of your physical, and the fantastical of your dreams, let's realize the foundation of what's to come IS ALREADY BUILT!

And let's continue to remember that JOY, PLAY, and FUN are our traveling companions as we move forward. But, really, BRAVO, my friend!

Now let's switch gears and move into a different realm, the one from which all things tangible germinate: OUR DREAMS. This is one of my favorite games, because it takes us right to the heart of the matter—that place that pumps life into every aspect of our being. This is the place that ultimately fuels what becomes our STYLE. Here the only limits are the ones we choose for ourselves. And in fact, it's a misnomer to call them limits. They are instead our INSPIRATIONS.

So, without further ado, we move into . . .

DON'T FENCE ME IN!

INSPIRATION, THE MOTHER OF YOUR STYLE

For your style to be authentic, it must originate from the center of your soul. It cannot start from anywhere outside of your deepest desires, or you are "borrowing" it from someone else. Deep inside each of us exists an endless universe of possibilities; I like to call this your *place of wonder.*

All you need to do is tap into this space to feel the power that resides there. It is the hub of our creativity. This is our core, and it is the source of both our DREAMS and our INSPIRATION, which are the wings upon which our soul flies through life!

Inspiration is the mother of your style. This is where your style is birthed, nurtured, and cultivated, until it develops into its unique form. This is also what makes it exclusive to you. Your inspiration is yours, and yours alone. No one else can lay a claim to it. That is why to be authentically yours, your style must always start there.

Inspiration comes from one place only: our DREAMS. Our dreams are where our heart and soul speak to us. It is their *language* we want to learn to listen to. When we follow our dreams, we are following our purpose and living our fullest life. We are also spreading JOY. We are tapping right into our place of wonder.

Our dreams are unlimited. They have no boundaries. But the surest way to deflate a dream is to try to put it in a box. When you don't allow your dreams to challenge the status quo, they wither and die. And likewise, when your style does not emanate from your dreams, it can never be truly yours.

So, I want you to get in touch with your core INSPIRATION by creating a DREAM BOARD. This is a collage of specific images that spring from your place of wonder and make your heart sing. This is going to be the core touchstone for your authentic style!

You'll do this on a scrapbook-type site such as Pinterest. I want you to search online for the one specific image that thrills you in each of the following categories:

1. **A BUILDING**

2. **A LANDSCAPE**

3. **A TREE**

4. **A FLOWER**

5. **A GARDEN**

6. **A SKY**

7. **A GOWN** (formal, any length)

8. **ANY IMAGE THAT DELIGHTS**

9. **ANOTHER IMAGE THAT DELIGHTS**

Now, the only criterion for this game is that each image makes you *tingle with* JOY. (If any of the items is not conducive to your sensibility, replace it. For example, maybe you aren't a garden person. If you want to do a beach or woods, etc., substitute. The only one that is not replaceable is the gown.)

Once you've amassed the collage, I want you to peruse it this way:

First, get centered by doing the three-step warm-up. (This is important so you can plug into your source in order to receive the full benefit this game provides.)

Then take in the entire collage as a whole. Check your reaction. If it doesn't transport you to your wonder place, find the weak link. Go over each image to check your reaction the same way. When you have every image aligned with your inspiration, it should be a source of delight and joy. *I want you to go for the tingle!*

We will use this later, as your standard for the starting point for creating specific outfits and a checkpoint for delineating the difference between what is Authentic to you or Imitative of others.

Remember, we only want to identify your place of INSPIRATION here. This is where your style becomes yours and yours alone! As I said, "Inspiration is the Mother of your Style." *Mamma mia!*

RECORD THE LINK TO YOUR COLLAGE HERE:

WHEN WE FOLLOW OUR DREAMS WE ARE FOLLOWING OUR PURPOSE— AND SPREADING JOY!

LET'S CHAT!

TIME FOR A "CUPPA"

Before we move into the next phase of our games, I'd like us to have a little "sit-down" so I can give you a glimpse of where we are headed as well as keep you from veering off into any detours.

So, pull up a chair; pour a cup of tea, coffee, or whatever beverage you like (although perhaps save the wine for a bit later!); and let's chat!

We're at the point now where we can start to get into a new type of understanding, what some people describe as the more tangible parts of our journey: IMAGE IDENTITIES, YIN/YANG BALANCE, and PERSONAL LINE AND SILHOUETTE.

But, like all the other parts of our DIY journey, they are actually just *pieces of the larger puzzle,* which is the emergence of your authentic style. None of these, by themselves, will take you to this ultimate destination.

Likewise, without the inspiring discoveries you've already made, this new phase would be lacking the depth of your complete self.

It's the combination of what you've previously gained paired with what we are about to undergo, concluding with what will follow, that will take you to that magic land that is your authentic style. Anything less would simply be, at its very best, *a pale façade of the rich and multidimensional celestial being you are*!

Basically, what I want to remind you of here is the importance of avoiding one of the major detours that are sure to misdirect you: YOU CAN'T PICK AND CHOOSE. Likewise, NO JUMPING AHEAD. You have to travel the entire path to get to your destination!

There is no shortcut to style. One does not, and cannot, exist. It's ALL of the galvanizing discoveries along the way that will ADD UP to what becomes your authentic style.

As we move forward, I will also help you untangle yourself from the myths and misinformation that can trap you into false assumptions.

So, let's raise our cup and salute your new chapter.

YOU HAVE TO TRAVEL THE ENTIRE PATH TO GET TO YOUR DESTINATION!

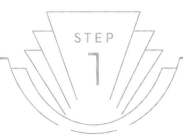

STEP

1

YOUR IMAGE IDENTITY

YOU'RE ENTITLED TO A TITLE!

Your story, as we've discovered so far, is spectacular! While we are still just midway through pinpointing the major components of it, look at how it's already unfolding!

It's filled with your dreams, your inspirations, your unique beauty, your potential, your history, your taste, your purpose—all those things we've explored and uncovered via playing the games! Just the experiences you've created so far have revealed such fabulous details about who you are!

Most of all, we've admitted that *you are stardust brought to life*! A one-of-a-kind "blazer" created to take your place among the illuminati that enlighten the world! Your story, even at this point, is a block-buster, a bestseller, a page-turner that anyone would be hard-pressed to put down!

So it stands to reason that a story as inimitable as yours deserves an equally definitive title. Your story needs a proper name! A title that is as unique as you!

YOUR IMAGE IDENTITY IS THAT NAME!

I created the entire IMAGE IDENTITY technique as a way to capture the heart and soul of your STYLE JOURNEY. It is designed to convey the very core of all you are and express it to both yourself and the world you inhabit, with *clarity and focus*.

It's like your personal gestalt: a composition that is more than the sum of your parts!

However, it's important to remember that the title of a story can come only AFTER that story is actually lived. *You can't start with a title*. It is designed to capture the gist of the story that is being told inside.

In other words, we have to discover and define more of the details that tell your fabulous story before we can give it a name!

This is why, while we are already a good ways into the content of your story, now we need to establish it more in physical terms before we can assign it the proper name. (We are looking to actually get dressed at some point, right?)

If your IMAGE IDENTITY is the identifica-tion of you, we need to understand how it literally manifests. We have to learn how your body and the clothes that will accentuate and elevate it intersect.

In other words: How do we dress your body?

Remember earlier when we discussed how style is an acquired skill? How even Fred Astaire didn't just leap out of the womb with top hat and tails?

We need a concrete technique that accurately defines your body in terms of how clothes actually work with its unique beauty. Your body is special; therefore, so must your clothes define it in that special way!

So—first your body, then your clothes!

ENNOBLE YOUR FORM

> *You only get one body; it is the temple of your soul.*
> —OLI HILLE

It is now time to begin work on your SCULPTURE. Later we'll come back to the related PAINTING. But first it's the stage of our journey where we are going to define and honor your perfect form!

MICHELANGELO AND YOU!

"I saw the angel in the marble and carved until I set him free. I simply carved away everything that was not David." (This was Michelangelo's reported response to being asked how he arrived at his masterwork.)

Now, let's agree, there's much more to a sculpture than just its outer form, but it's through that physical form that its soul gets voiced.

Likewise, you certainly are more than just your body. Yet, it's that very body of yours that is your soul's mouthpiece.

Later in our adventure, we'll spend a good amount of time learning how to express your inner self through *Situation* and *Intent*. Right now, we are going to start with your framework.

Your sculpture contains everything you are—your inner angel and your outer masterpiece. So this part of our quest becomes: *How do we harmoniously honor your sculpture?*

First, we have to DEFINE your sculpture. Then we have to learn how to WORK IN HARMONY with it.

There are the same two parts that also will determine your Image Identity:

1. **YOUR YIN/YANG BALANCE (FOR DEFINITION).** This is how we are going to describe your sculpture.

2. **YOUR PERSONAL LINE (FOR MANIFESTATION).** This is the blueprint for building your sculpture.

It is the discovery of both that determines your IMAGE IDENTITY.

Now, I realize you are eager to get to the actual determination of your personal Image Identity. (Believe me, so am I!) In just a bit, we are going to do exactly that! I am going to have it all charted out and also illustrated for you!

But in order for me to get you there, we need to understand these two fundamentals we are using to define you.

So, let's do a deeper dive into each!

THE YIN AND THE YANG OF IT ALL

DEFINING YOUR DESIGN

> *The relationship between Yin and Yang is that of a partnership. The universe would be impossible without their interaction.*
>
> —JOHN B. COBB

> *It takes two to Tao.*
>
> —ANA CLAUDIA ANTUNES

We have to find a way to help you understand what kind of sculpture you are. How are the parts of you put together in one whole composition? Are you Art Deco sleek and chic? Maybe a Grecian goddess? Perhaps you are exuberantly rococo? What is the unique beauty that is integral to your unique concoction?

Seeing yourself from a little distance by learning a technique so you'll be able to accept and pay tribute to your unique magnum opus is key. You need a method that will identify your frame and also teach you how to work in harmony with it.

The solution to this is my adaptation of the ancient Chinese philosophy of YIN and YANG.

Yin and Yang is the realization of the CONTRAST OF OPPOSITES in Nature that defines our world.

Now, in a bit we are going to translate your sculpture onto my yin/yang scale, which will take us to your Image Identity and the land of your line! But before we get there, let's take a moment to explore: What exactly is this yin-and-yang thing all about?

To illustrate in abstract terms:

LET'S HAVE A LITTLE FUN!

YIN	YANG		YIN	YANG
Short—	Tall		Rococo—	Art Deco
Circular—	Sharp		Victorian—	Cubism
Moon—	Sun		Chopin—	Stravinsky
Valley—	Mountain		Rose—	Calla Lily

Now of course, these are generalities, but I think you get the picture. We can translate anything onto the yin/yang scale. More important, regardless of your personal taste, there is exquisite beauty to be found and celebrated in all areas of both opposites.

The other thing about yin/yang that's so vital to your specific journey is that it's also based on recognizing the interdependency of these polar extremes as critical to life.

In other words, we can't have yin without yang. There is no one without the other.

The only way we can comprehend short is to understand tall. There is no moon without the sun. We can't have a valley unless we also have a mountain. How would we define curves without angles? Everything we experience and understand is completely dependent on our acceptance of CONTRAST.

The most beautiful thing about this, from my perspective, and the most important for our purposes, is that there is no judgment in either extreme.

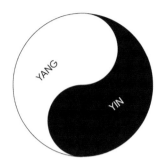

YIN YANG: THE EXTREMES

They are both honored as essential to our life. Each is seen as exceptional and beautiful in its singular attributes.

This is why the symbol of yin/yang is circular, not linear. It ends where it begins. The two halves combine to make one whole.

So, what does this mean for us? Well, to begin with, let's play a little!

YOUR PRESENCE IS REQUESTED

THE YIN/YANG FESTIVITIES

I want to invite you to join me in the celebration of the beauty of the yin and the majesty of the yang. We are going to make merry as we explore and expand your appreciation of both sides of the spectrum before we translate your sculpture onto it.

So we are going to play the next two games now.

They are both going to do two things simultaneously, *while you are playing them*! One is to help you see and rejoice in both extremes of the yin and the yang. The other is, at the same time, going to help you identify where your prejudices are, both positive and negative.

SEE IT, FEEL IT, RECORD IT!

Create two collages on a scrapbook site (such as Pinterest), one for yin, one for yang, with six images in each collage. They can be literal or abstract. Just make sure they are **YOUR PERSONAL** ideas of both extremes. (You can refer back to the list on page 57 where I identified yin and yang examples, or simply use any ideas you personally relate to.) It's not necessary for you to like these images. At this point, we just want to identify your perception of them.

After you have created these two collages, make notes about your emotional reaction to *each separate image* in both collections. **WRITE THESE DOWN.**

Do they make you smile? Do they make you feel uneasy? There is **NO JUDGMENT** here, it's just to help you recognize your reflexive response to each. The goal for this is simply to identify your own idea of each extreme and to observe your emotional "knee-jerk" response to each.

(This last step will prove to be crucial later, as we move into identifying your specific place on the yin/yang scale and how that translates into all your personal style details.)

RECORD YOUR REACTIONS TO YOUR COLLAGES HERE:

Positive reactions:

_____

_____

_____

_____

Negative reactions:

_____

_____

_____

_____

At this point, you now will have a chance to move on to the appreciation and celebration of each extreme with . . .

YOUR YIN/YANG SOIREES

PARTYIN' WITH YOUR PEEPS!

Now I'd like YOU to invite us to help you paint the town red with two spectacular yin/yang shindigs! Your yin gala and your yang bash are sure to be the hottest tickets of the season!

So please create two more collages on your scrapbook site: a combination of the most delightful yin images and the most delightful yang images you can come up with connected to festivities that you would adore to create! These should be two different types of whatever parties would float your boat; just make sure that they are both delicious and totally beguiling to you.

One might choose something like a garden party with its florals and fripperies for one collage. Someone else's board could be a cozy movie night for a select few intimates.

It doesn't matter how elaborate or simple they are; it's just YOUR version of two different delightful events, chosen to represent your personal vision of either extreme. (Remember, this is playtime, totally imaginary—so there is no limit in budget, décor, attire, or location. Feel free to travel to the decade or even century of your heart's desire!)

After you've created both, write down a brief description of each.

Note: Do not underestimate the value of this game. As we have previously discussed, both JOY and ASPIRATION are the parts of your style that make it authentically and uniquely yours. These are elements that YOU and ONLY YOU bring to your style. Elucidating them is not simply important, it is KEY.

Here's a bit of frivolous fun, as an example:

(Now, you have to remember, I grew up in a small town in the Midwest, believing that everyone in the city lived in penthouses and went dancing all night long! Boy, was I surprised!)

LET'S GO NIGHTCLUBBING

EXTREME YANG

The decade: 1920s. The Cotton Club. Lena Horne encased in slinky silver sequins, torching on the black lacquer stage. The smoking-hot jazz of Duke Ellington steams up the dance floor while flappers lean on tables swilling bootleg hooch. Fringe reigns and beaded headgear is the cat's meow!

EXTREME YIN

The decade: 1950s. It's a balmy moonlit night in Hollywood and the Cocoanut Grove is packed. Marilyn Monroe and Elizabeth Taylor are vying for best décolleté while Johnny Mathis croons away in a creamy white dinner jacket. It's bubbly champagne and fragrant gardenias on every table while movie stars swirl around the palm-fringed dance floor in mounds of tulle.

Whether you dream of bonfires, après ski, beach bashes, or tea party finery is no matter at all. I just want you to go all out with whatever toots your horn!

"JOY!"

RECORD A BRIEF DESCRIPTION OF YOUR TWO SOIREES HERE:

Your Yin Soiree description

_____

_____

_____

Your Yang Soiree description

_____

_____

_____

Now that we've got a handle on the ethos of yin and yang and expanded your appreciation of the specific beauty of each, let's direct them a bit more toward how we define your frame and how to drape it!

NOTE: As we move forward into this phase, it's important that you are not yet trying to figure out what you are. We will get there, I promise! Just stay with me as we explore the extremes. We are learning technique here, not defining you. (Let me refer back to my piano training with you for a moment. Before we can play Rachmaninoff, we have to do our finger exercises!)

FIRST UP, THE EXTREMES

SYNCHRONICITY FOR COMPLICITY

Now, let's not start pretending this is complicated here! How about we take a moment to touch base again and remember the one basic tenet of this entire system: WORKING IN HARMONY WITH NATURE.

It's really simple: First, we define you, then we drape you harmoniously. Then we give it a name that helps you focus the entire gestalt of you!

Don't let anyone or anything mess you up about this! When in doubt, simply go back to this one idea: Follow what nature set out for you!

Keep this front and center and you'll never falter. So, let's take a look at how yin/yang fulfills this.

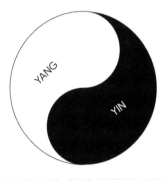

YIN YANG: THE EXTREMES

YANG EXTREME	YIN EXTREME
PHYSICAL:	PHYSICAL:
Sharp, Narrow, Elongated	Curved, Soft, Elliptical
CLOTHING:	CLOTHING:
Tailored, Sleek	Flowing, Shapely
EXAMPLE:	EXAMPLE:
Katharine Hepburn	Elizabeth Taylor

Now, don't forget at this point: We are NOT talking about YOU. We are just practicing our understanding of the craft.

THE ARCHETYPES

SYMBOLS, NOT PEOPLE!

I created a joining of the yin/yang philosophy with the archetypal prototypes to provide an authentic connection between you and your body that moves past your subjective prejudices. This is the heart of that *intelligent subjectivity* we are in the midst of achieving!

The Archetypes are merely generic symbols.

You are not an Archetype (or any kind of type!). You are a PERSON, an INDIVIDUAL. Ultimately, we will define you by both your IMAGE IDENTITY, and how your PERSONAL LINE is expressed. That is coming!

For now, let's get clearer on the five Archetypes and where they fall in the yin/yang universe.

ARCHETYPE YIN/YANG PLACEMENT

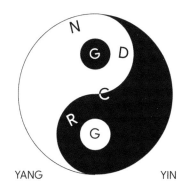

YANG   YIN

YIN YANG: 5 ARCHETYPES

DRAMATIC:
Extreme, sharp yang (narrow, elongated)

ROMANTIC:
Extreme, soft yin (lush, curvaceous)

CLASSIC:
Evenly balanced between extremes (symmetrical)

NATURAL:
Yang (blunt, soft-edged)

GAMINE:
Combination of opposites (yin in size, yang in frame)

NOTE: There are no celebrity examples here because, once again: PEOPLE ARE NOT ARCHETYPES.

Where do we go from here? Well, let's first identify the actual IMAGE IDENTITY THEMES. After that we will find out how they relate to you specifically.

FROM ARCHETYPE TO IMAGE IDENTITY

THE ZEN OF THE TEN

The five archetypes are allegorical. They are symbols. Symbols can give us an instant reference when words alone are too complicated. But for us, they are not specific to you as a person. This is why we must only use them as generic *influences* to help us utilize the polar extremes they represent.

What I mean by that is, you are not an ARCHETYPE. You are not a type of any kind. That would be turning you into a stereotype, another version of a preconceived box to force you into.

What we want to do is borrow the generic starting point of the Archetypes and make it specific to YOU. This is called your IMAGE IDENTITY. Ultimately, there are ten possibilities.

Your IMAGE IDENTITY is simply the name that describes your specific place on the yin/yang scale. Later, we will learn how you as an individual materialize that into your style.

For now, once again, please, please, please—*do not try to figure out "what you are" or how these apply to you*. Let's just learn the ten Identities and their placement in terms of yin and yang. I promise we'll unpack these in much greater detail at further stops along our journey. At this point, it's simply about clarifying the process so we can ultimately find your own Image Identity.

THE DRAMATICS

DRAMATIC
YANG, extreme sharp

SOFT DRAMATIC
YANG, with a pronounced yin undercurrent

THE ROMANTICS

ROMANTIC
YIN, extreme soft

THEATRICAL ROMANTIC
YIN, with a yang undercurrent

THE CLASSICS

DRAMATIC CLASSIC
BALANCED, with yang influence

SOFT CLASSIC
BALANCED, with yin influence

THE NATURALS

FLAMBOYANT NATURAL
YANG, bold blunt

SOFT NATURAL
YANG with a yin undercurrent

THE GAMINES

FLAMBOYANT GAMINE
COMBO OF OPPOSITES, extra yang

SOFT GAMINE
COMBO OF OPPOSITES, extra yin

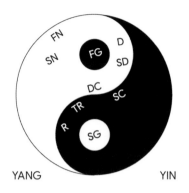

YIN YANG: 10 IMAGE IDENTITIES

Now that we've gotten a general idea of the concept of yin/yang, let's move into the second piece of what determines your IMAGE IDENTITY: the part that actually manifests in today's clothes: *YOUR PERSONAL LINE and how it connects to SILHOUETTE.*

To understand why your PERSONAL LINE is a prerequisite to your IMAGE IDENTITY, you have to first learn about its connection to SILHOUETTE. This is why the concept of PERSONAL LINE exists in the first place!

Now, this is going to be something you haven't heard of before, because I created it based on the radical change in the way clothing is constructed that has occurred in the last decades. So we'll go step by step.

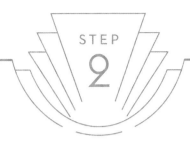

PERSONAL LINE & SILHOUETTE

THIS PAIR IS NOT A "PEAR"!

Your PERSONAL LINE is based on how the *proportions* of your body relate to each other in *one long outline*.

A SILHOUETTE is the outline of an outfit *as it's worn on your body*. It is the COMBINATION of outfit and you in *one unbroken shape*.

This is a very simple concept:

Your SILHOUETTE needs to ACCOMMODATE your PERSONAL LINE.
(This is called creating a *Complementary Silhouette*)

Your PERSONAL LINE could be described as: THE BLUEPRINT FOR YOUR SILHOUETTE.

Now, it's imperative that you don't conflate "line" with "body type," "body parts," "fruit shapes," or any other old ideas that start with a preconceived shape or box that requires you to be fit into. Your PERSONAL LINE is NOT something predetermined you are going to be *forced into*. It's specific to the way nature has laid out *your individual form*.

The reason it's so crucial to replace these outdated ideas on shapes and types with this new concept is because of the way silhouettes have been *fundamentally transformed by today's fabrics and designs*.

To understand why this is an essential difference, let's delve into what today's silhouettes actually require.

FRUITS ARE FOR SALAD! YOU ARE NOT A KUMQUAT!

SILHOUETTE RULES!

> *The eye has to travel.*
>
> —DIANA VREELAND

First, let's reiterate: SILHOUETTE is *the outline of a garment as it's worn on the body.* It's one long unbroken line that travels around the shape of the outfit as you have it on (not on the hanger). It's important to understand that on the female form, clothes: 1) HANG off the shoulders, and 2) DRAPE around the curves (bust and hips).

Since our guiding motivation is working in harmony with nature, our goal is to discover how to create a SILHOUETE that is *complementary* to your body's PERSONAL LINE.

This is critical to developing your authentic style because silhouette is the initial visual statement of your unique beauty. It's your first line of communication of who you are and what you are about!

When someone looks at us, the first thing the eye does is travel around our SHAPE. It's what the eye and brain simultaneously take in, instantaneously!

So, if we want our style to be truly authentic, we need harmony between outfit and self. (Again, ultimately, we look to include more than just our body, but right now, the body is our starting point.)

FROM TOGAS TO FLAPPERS

DRESSING IS HISTORY'S SHOWCASE

Here's where a bit of history helps us understand why a new approach was necessary, and why I was led to create this entirely new technique. Historically, a silhouette was constructed *outside the body.* It existed on its own, irrelevant to the body that would be wearing it. Clothes were built as if they were "stand-alones." The body was meant either to be covered over or forced into whatever silhouette was popular.

This primarily required construction, tailoring, and underpinnings to create an *independent silhouette that was very strictly defined.* The result was that you had to shoehorn yourself into a *preconceived silhouette.*

This also meant a lot of foundation undergarments were required in order to fit you into the preconstructed garment. The false "wasp waist" that was created by corsets and waist cinchers is the most obvious example of this. Even when corsets were beginning to disappear in the 1920s and '30s, the silhouette was still a pre-conscribed shape.

During these eras, silhouettes were also decreed periodically, handed down from the designers as well as being influenced by world events. This is the reason we used to be able to define a decade by its definitive silhouette.

The History of Silhouette being connected to the changing mores of the times goes back thousands

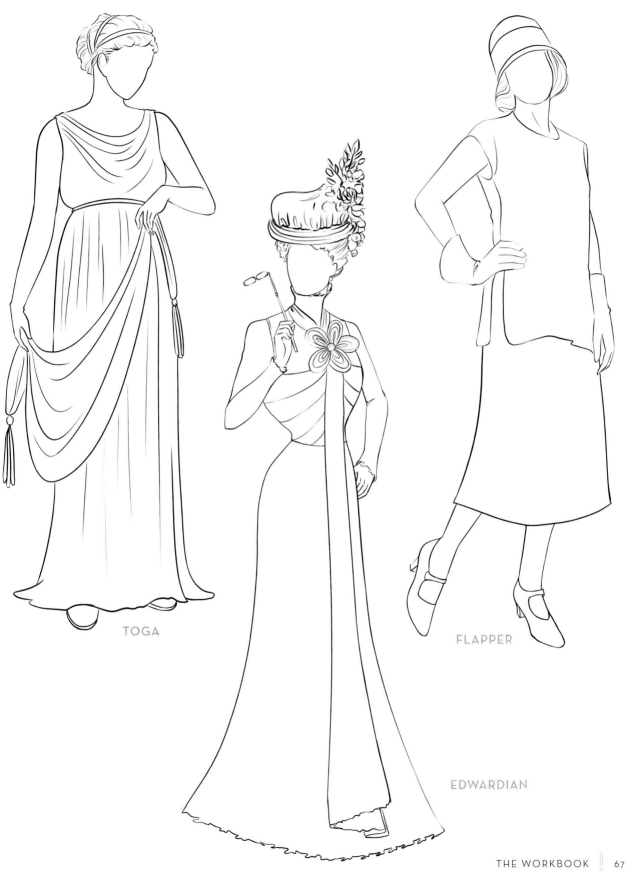

TOGA

EDWARDIAN

FLAPPER

of years! Society's environments, from long before ancient Egypt through modern times, had always been the catalyst for what we could define as the *silhouette of the era*. You only need to go back to the middle of the twentieth century for the two most distinct examples of our time.

World War II was a period of unity of purpose and shared sacrifice. The resulting silhouette that defined the 1940s reflected the desire to show solidarity along with the need for austerity. This was the genesis of the upside-down triangle shape created by powered shoulders and a slimmed-down body.

Two years after the war ended, in 1947, Christian Dior captured the world's sigh of relief and need for celebration with his New Look silhouette. Waspwaisted and padded hips; these were the visual repudiation of the rationing and struggle of the war years. It was like the visual after-party of the previous darker times that became the hallmark of the 1950s.

The point of both, however, was that they were each the one defining look that every woman was shown. These were both strong shapes that were constructed outside the body. You were told to fit yourself into these, whatever your body was created to be. Hence, the rules and restrictions of the so-called body types that were designed to force you into these silhouettes were born!

Variations of this idea of the preconstructed silhouette continued for most of the twentieth century, until the 1980s, when there emerged something that changed this idea forever!

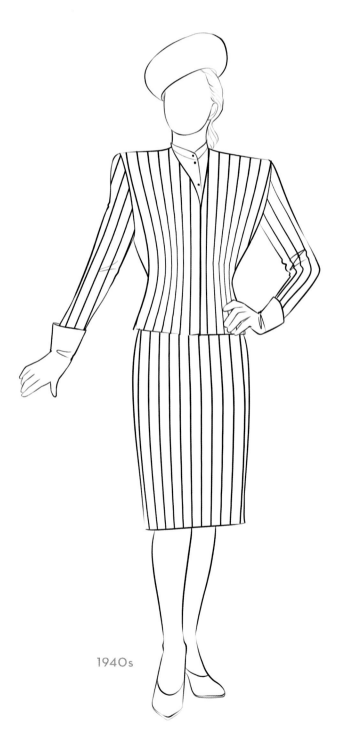

1940s

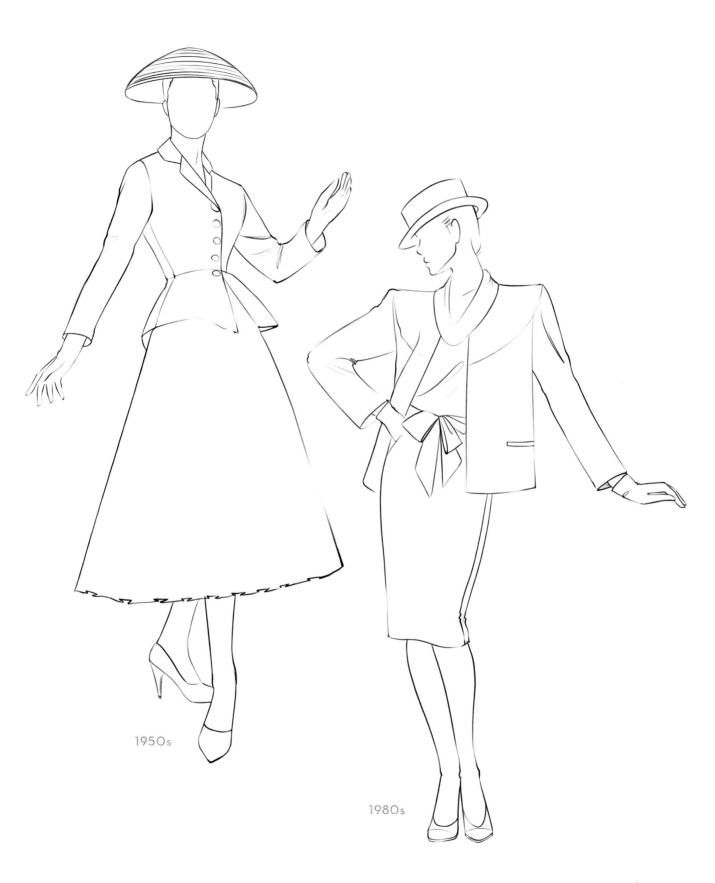

1950s

1980s

SEA CHANGE BY FABRIC!

IT'S ALL ABOUT THE STRETCH

In the mideighties, I was in a meeting with two representatives of a major shoe designer who were looking to partner with me on the launch of a new product they were going to be introducing to the United States with much fanfare.

What they had laid out on my desk (and were actually also wearing!) was this new item—pantyhose with LYCRA. (It was the Lycra that would prove to be the game-changer, not the pantyhose!) Stretch in fabric was going to become the new norm in the next twenty years.

Fast-forward to today, and we find that stretch in fabric has totally upended the very nature and creation of silhouette. The flexibility and lighter weight of this modern fabric hangs and drapes entirely differently than fabric did before it was utilized.

Today, instead of a preconstructed silhouette that exists outside the body, *a garment must interact with the body* to create a silhouette. That means it's a COMBINATION of body and garment that creates a modern silhouette.

This is why a completely different way of approaching COMPLEMENTARY CLOTHING is necessary.

FRUITS ARE FOR SALAD—YOU ARE NOT A KUMQUAT!

HARMONY, NOT SYMMETRY

In the older times, the "rules" were all based on that shoehorning idea of coercing your body into the outfit. Since the silhouette was already formed, you were given requirements of how to refigure your body to conform to what was already created by the garment/outfit.

The most concrete example was the fruits. For example: You are a "pear" (which meant your hips are big), so you need to add to your top to "balance" the outfit.

This was because, with all the earlier clothing, the so-called ideal standard of these rules used *symmetry* as the goal.

Since no one is actually symmetrical, these rules and "types" were manufactured to CREATE THE ILLUSION OF SYMMETRY. That means they started with the concept that you are less than perfect, and you needed these "types" to correct that.

I always have rejected this idea, as it goes against everything Love-Based Beauty stands for. Instead of starting with the "less than" concept, my technique has always promoted WORKING IN HARMONY WITH YOUR NATURAL PROPORTIONS.

Love-Based Beauty has also proven to be the only way that today's revised silhouettes can actually be achieved. The fabric of today doesn't form in that same old preconstructed way. Your body is its own perfect template for this new silhouette.

If you try to "balance your apple," you will eliminate 90 percent of the amazing possibilities that exist in clothing stores! You will also erase the very things that are special and unique about you. The clothes of today just don't work that way!

Today, the old body types can't allow for all the fabulous diversity of clothing, design, and beauty that we seek to both take advantage of and honor.

So today, no fruits, no body types, and no balancing-out rules. Instead, I want you to learn to . . .

HONOR YOUR LINE

YOUR BODY AS THE PERFECT FIGURE

What we are going to do now is define YOUR PERSONAL LINE. In order to do that, you've got to "put on a new pair of eyeglasses."

Now, this is different from the way you view and define silhouette. Silhouette is a simple shape of the outfit as it's being worn. It's direct. You get what you see.

You can't simply look at your body to see your PERSONAL LINE. It doesn't show up that way. *It's something you have to learn.*

Your PERSONAL LINE is all about PROPORTION. It's based on how your individual pieces relate to each other in *one long outline.*

It's not about how they look to you as you gaze at your body. *In fact, you* CANNOT *see your Personal Line by looking directly at your figure.* It's not there to be seen. Instead of "seeing" it, we have to DEFINE it.

Remember when we spoke before about the fact that clothes hang off the shoulders and drape around the contours of the figure? *The way your body requires this to occur is what defines your* PERSONAL LINE.

To make that clear-cut and workable for you, I've devised this technique that defines your Personal Line in simple terms.

We will first learn how fabric would hang and drape on your specific form (your sculpture). Then we will assign the descriptive tags that will DEFINE YOUR PERSONAL LINE.

Your Personal Line will then teach you what you need to accommodate in a complementary silhouette.

The beauty of this technique is that not only is it required for today's clothes, it allows you total freedom. Once you learn what your Personal Line requires, there are a multitude of ways you can express that.

Silhouette is flexible today. It allows for however many "looks" you are excited to create! That is why understanding your Personal Line is indispensable to today's styles. It's also why the old body types, fruits, etc. simply don't fit into what today's fashions offer!

NO FRUITS, NO BODY TYPES, AND NO "BALANCING-OUT" RULES.

ALIGN WITH YOUR LINE!

YOU ARE EXACTLY WHO YOU ARE "SUPPOSED" TO BE!

Since this is a new technique and has never been put out before, let's spend a bit more time getting familiar with its meaning and its purpose.

I devised this entire method for one basic reason: to give you a simple and direct way to harness this totally re-formed silhouette of today and make it work for you!

Because the old ways are just not applicable, I knew it was imperative to come up with a way that would work in our DIY approach. You have to be able to define this for yourself. You can't rely on misadvice from either old ways or internet myths. It has to be personal to you and totally opposite of the generic "type" approach that puts you in a box.

The biggest stumbling block is that *you can't "see" your line on your body.* It's a template that you use to create a complementary silhouette. *It doesn't exist on your body.* You have to devise it. (There are no "lines" on your body or on clothes. That's another *internet misguide.*)

LET ME REITERATE THE TWO SIMPLE PREMISES FOR LINE AND SILHOUETTE:

1. Your PERSONAL LINE is a blueprint for creating a COMPLEMENTARY SILHOUETTE.

2. Your SILHOUETTE needs to accommodate your PERSONAL LINE.

The reason for a blueprint for anything is to be the *outline* for what you are going to build. It gives you the underlying framework to complete a design. *You can't construct a building without first creating a blueprint!*

So, the question then becomes: "*What does your individual blueprint require to create a complementary silhouette for you, individually?*"

It requires the understanding of what your specific body needs in a silhouette in order for your clothes to hang and drape properly.

In other words, how do clothes hang/drape on your specific sculpture?

This will come from your discovering the RATIO of how the individual parts of your body fit together. It's the proportions of how the parts of your body relate to each other that count.

It's NOT the individual body parts by themselves. It's the *sum total of the whole* as defined by ONE LONG LINE. This is what's required of your Silhouette to accommodate.

We can figure this out by looking at how fabric hangs down from the shoulders and drapes around the body.

Let me give you two examples:

I'm going to start with a piece of *imaginary fabric* (a sheer silk chiffon, weighted at the bottom) and drape it down from the shoulders. Then we will see where it either hangs down straight along the body or where the body pushes it out.

If the fabric were to hang straight down from the shoulders in one long line, we can determine you have what we will call a VERTICAL LINE and will then need a VERTICAL SILHOUETTE *that hangs straight down your body.*

On the other hand, if the fabric is pushed out by your bust, cuts inward in the middle, and is pushed out and around again by your hips, then we can determine you have what we will call a CURVED LINE and will need a CURVED SILHOUETTE that drapes around the curves of your body.

Remember as you view this, THIS IS NOT AN OUTLINE OF THE BODY. It also is NOT FABRIC STRETCHED AROUND THE BODY. It skims the body, floating down from the shoulders.

Take a look at the two different bodies illustrated below. The actual body is outlined in black. The red outline is the how the imaginary fabric would hang/drape on the body. (In a moment, we will learn to call this your DOMINANT.)

Now, remember, when I first introduced yin and yang, we started by simply learning about the CONCEPT. *Do not try to figure out what you are at this point.* After we go through the next game, we will pinpoint your PERSONAL LINE.

For now, can you just see how this works in the illustration?

It's pretty straightforward. Once again, this is based on WORKING IN HARMONY with YOU! We simply want *a Silhouette that's in harmony with your Sculpture!*

It's the technique I invented so you can translate the way clothes and your body can make beautiful music together!

To do this, we need to create your LINE SKETCH! This will be a simple line you superimpose on a photo.

Now, everyone has both one DOMINANT and one ADDITIONAL to define their LINE. So, let's start with the DOMINANT, which we will call either VERTICAL or CURVE, just like in the example and illustration below.

THE DOMINANTS

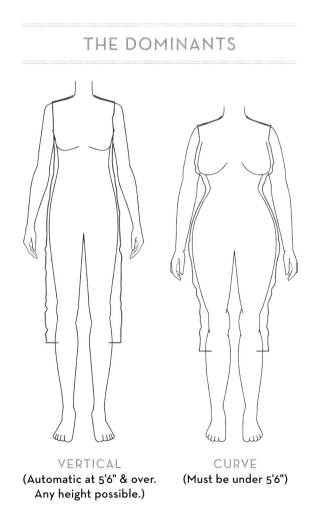

VERTICAL
(Automatic at 5'6" & over.
Any height possible.)

CURVE
(Must be under 5'6")

WHAT'S MY LINE?

PART ONE: DEFINE YOUR DOMINANT

First, I am going to ask you to take a photo of yourself. Then you are going to superimpose a sketch of how the "imaginary fabric" falls on your photo. (You can either do this on your computer or print the photo and do it on the printout.)

Don't get nervous! It's very simple. Just follow the instructions and you will have it done in no time!

First, you need a clear, unobstructed image of your body in form-fitting clothes. A leotard and tights, a swimsuit, or close-fitting undergarments will be perfect.

Now, standing in a relaxed, neutral pose, take a full-length photo, full frontal, from about ten feet away, at chest height. Let your arms hang straight down at your sides and keep your feet about three inches apart. Either use your phone camera or, if you prefer, have a friend take this. **(DO NOT DO THIS IN A MIRROR.)**

Next, you simply want to do the exact same thing I showed you on the illustrations of **VERTICAL** and **CURVE** above.

You're going to see how the *imaginary fabric of silk chiffon weighted at the bottom* will either hang straight down from your shoulder or gets pushed out and around the flesh of your body.

So, on your photo, starting at the edge of the shoulder where it meets the upper arm, let the "fabric" fall down. Whether it hangs straight down or whether the bust/hip area pushes the "fabric" out and around them is what you want to sketch.

NOTE: It is crucial here to repeat what was previously noted: **This is NOT an outline of your body.** We are looking **ONLY** to see where your body pushes the imaginary fabric out or does not. The "fabric," being silk chiffon, *skims* the body. **It is NOT a form-fitting line.**

The fabric will either do one or the other. It will either *hang straight down from the shoulder* **OR** be *pushed out and around by the bust/hips.* Then it is up to you to simply **REPORT** what your sketch shows.

If the line moves relatively straight down, your dominant is **VERTICAL**. If it got pushed out by the bust and hip, your dominant is **CURVE**.

NOTE: *DO NOT REFER TO YOUR BODY OR YOUR BODY PARTS HERE. ONLY REPORT WHAT IS SHOWN BY THE SKETCH ITSELF.*

Remember, the point of this is to learn what you need to accommodate in a complementary silhouette.

If you will once again refer to the illustration on page 73, you can see how each of the two extremes is then accommodated by the appropriate clothing silhouette.

IF YOU ARE 5'6" or over, you are an automatic **VERTICAL**. (If you drew curves, that *may* be your **ADDITIONAL**, but for now you need to identify your dominant as **VERTICAL**.) There are no exceptions to *this*. (I'll explain more in detail farther along.) You may also have **VERTICAL** at any height under five foot six.

To have **CURVE** as your dominant, you must be under five foot six—though it is not automatic at this height, but you may not be over this height to have **CURVE** as your *dominant*.

(Remember that the height requirements are there to save you time and mistakes. This is about defining your **PERSONAL LINE**. It has nothing to do with how you think you appear or what is considered tall, short, or anything in between.)

MY DOMINANT IS (Check One)**:**   VERTICAL _____   CURVE _____

PART TWO: DEFINE YOUR ADDITIONAL

Your **PERSONAL LINE** will be a combination of **YOUR DOMINANT** plus **ONE ADDITIONAL**.

Now that we know your dominant, we need to define the second piece of your **PERSONAL LINE**, which is as important. This is your **ADDITIONAL**, which is what makes it specific to **YOU**!

Let me first identify and define the terms for your **SECONDARY**. Here is an illustration along with the definition of each. The red outline reiterates your **DOMINANT**, while the **ADDITIONAL** is outlined in the blue superimposed on the red as well as the area labeled where it occurs. Note that blue both has the area involved outlined as well as is pointed out with dots and arrows to show you clearly **EXACTLY** where the **SECONDARY** occurs on the body. (This area outlined is the **ONLY** area affected by your **SECONDARY**.)

CURVE (AS ADDITIONAL): Elliptical (oval) line, cutting in at midsection.

MODERATE: Parity between outer edge of the upper torso and hipbone. These two parts are evenly spaced.

WIDTH: Breadth through shoulder/upper torso area. This will be wider than what comes underneath. (It is proportionate. *It is not a wide body.* This part of the body is simply broader than the rest. You could be tiny and still have this part be wider.)

NARROW: Everything starts inward from the shoulder and moves down. (It may either go straight down or push out and around, but it stays within the shoulder line.)

DOUBLE CURVE: Two ellipses (ovals), bust and hips stacked on top of each other, with a definite indentation cutting inward between the two.

PETITE: Compact overall. Vertical or Curve packed within a compressed frame.

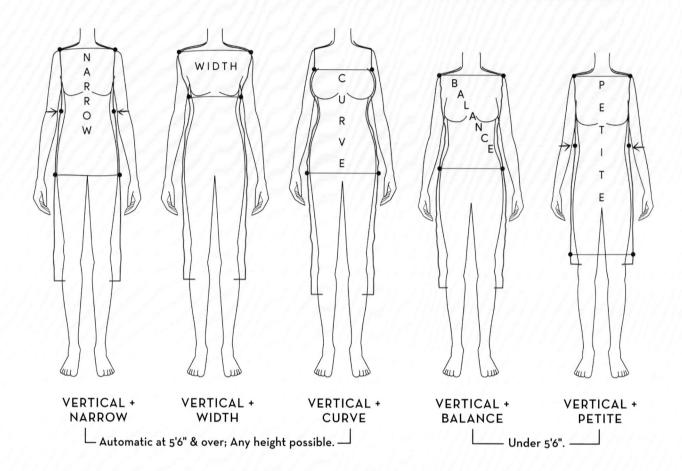

VERTICAL +
NARROW

VERTICAL +
WIDTH

VERTICAL +
CURVE

VERTICAL +
BALANCE

VERTICAL +
PETITE

Automatic at 5'6" & over; Any height possible.

Under 5'6".

Your PERSONAL LINE *will be a combination of* YOUR DOMINANT *plus* ONE ADDITIONAL.

Now, don't make this complicated. We already know one of your LINE pieces. All we have to do is determine the second piece!

Go back to the photo you took along with the LINE that determined your dominant. Using the illustrations and definitions above, sketch your additional line on your photo.

At this point your PERSONAL LINE SKETCH should most clearly resemble one of the illustrations on pages 78 and 79.

After you've done this, record your findings below. (NOTE: Only report what your sketch shows. Do not look at the photo of your body. It's ONLY the line sketch you've drawn that gives you the correct answer.)

THE CURVES + ADDITIONAL

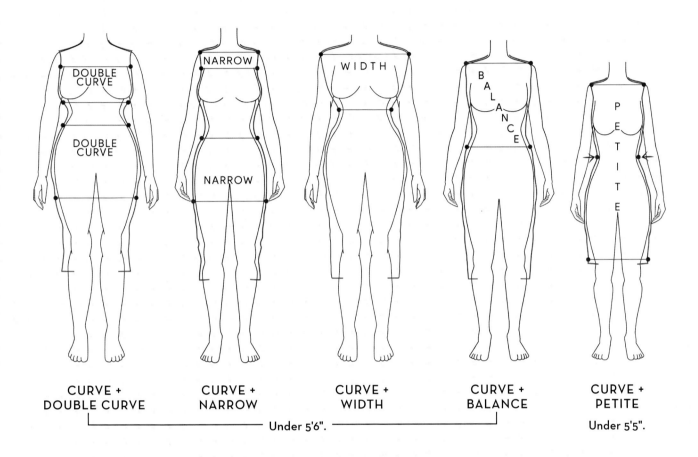

| CURVE + DOUBLE CURVE | CURVE + NARROW | CURVE + WIDTH | CURVE + BALANCE | CURVE + PETITE |

Under 5'6".

Under 5'5".

MY ADDITIONAL IS (Check One): CURVE _____   MODERATE _____
WIDTH _____   NARROW _____   DOUBLE CURVE _____   PETITE _____

(NOTE: Vertical cannot occur as an Additional.)
Now go back and retrieve your Dominant and record this along with what you've just identified as your Additional below. The combination (DOMINANT plus ADDITIONAL) is what you now can designate as your PERSONAL LINE!

A reminder: If you are five foot six or over, you have an automatic VERTICAL as your dominant. To have CURVE as your dominant, you must be under five foot six. (It is possible to be under five foot six and still have VERTICAL as your dominant.)

PART THREE: DEFINE YOUR PERSONAL LINE SKETCH

Here is an illustration of what your **PERSONAL LINE SKETCH SHOULD LOOK LIKE.** *(Remember that your red line is imaginary fabric, a soft, lightweight fabric like a silk chiffon, weighted down at the bottom. It skims the body; it is not simply an outline. Note that the red line is willowy.)*

YOUR PERSONAL LINE SKETCH: *Vertical + Additional*

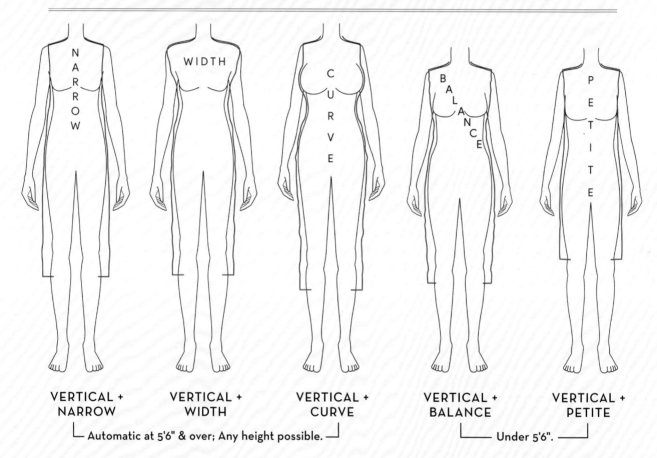

VERTICAL + NARROW	VERTICAL + WIDTH	VERTICAL + CURVE	VERTICAL + BALANCE	VERTICAL + PETITE

Automatic at 5'6" & over; Any height possible.   Under 5'6".

From now on, this is the sketch that you will always use as your **PERSONAL LINE,** that you will use as your reference for creating **COMPLEMENTARY SILHOUETTES.**

HIP HIP HOORAY, WE'VE DONE IT!!

We've done it! Congratulations! By traveling step by step, we've discovered all the pieces of your puzzle, and now we simply will put them together! *You are going to now be your own personal Michelangelo and release the inner angel that is* **YOU!**

Remember, your Image Identity is not a "type"! It's not a body type, not a personality type, or an essence/vibe. *It's the gestalt of your sculpture!*

And as I mentioned earlier, the nature of a sculpture is to be the mouthpiece that pronounces

YOUR PERSONAL LINE SKETCH: *Curve + Additional*

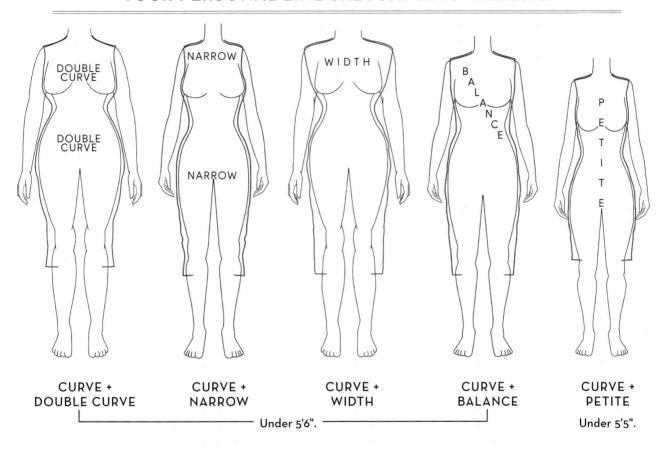

CURVE +
DOUBLE CURVE

CURVE +
NARROW

CURVE +
WIDTH

CURVE +
BALANCE

CURVE +
PETITE

— Under 5'6". —

Under 5'5".

MY PERSONAL LINE IS (Check One):

VERTICAL + NARROW _____

VERTICAL + CURVE _____

VERTICAL + BALANCE _____

VERTICAL + WIDTH _____

VERTICAL + PETITE _____

CURVE + DOUBLE CURVE _____

CURVE + NARROW _____

CURVE + BALANCE _____

CURVE + WIDTH _____

CURVE + PETITE _____

your unique beauty to the world! It's your vehicle for your dreams.

There are two pieces necessary to define your **IMAGE IDENTITY**, your **PERSONAL LINE** plus your **YIN/YANG BALANCE**. It's the combination of the latter two that determines the former.

You'll recall that in "The Zen of the Ten" (page 63),

I translated each Image Identity onto the yin/yang scale.

By discovering your **PERSONAL LINE**, we have, at the same time, determined your **YIN/YANG BALANCE**. Your Balance is your Line translated onto the Yin/Yang scale. It's already done!

So, without further ado, here you are!

IMAGE IDENTITY + YOUR YIN/YANG BALANCE + YOUR PERSONAL LINE

DRAMATIC	YANG, extreme sharp	Vertical + Narrow
SOFT DRAMATIC	YANG, with a pronounced yin undercurrent	Vertical + Curve
ROMANTIC	YIN, extreme soft	Curve + Double Curve
THEATRICAL ROMANTIC	YIN, with a yang undercurrent	Curve + Narrow
DRAMATIC CLASSIC	BALANCED, with a yang influence	Vertical + Balance
SOFT CLASSIC	BALANCED, with a yin influence	Curve + Balance
FLAMBOYANT NATURAL	YANG, bold, blunt	Vertical + Width
SOFT NATURAL	YANG, with a yin undercurrent	Curve + Width
FLAMBOYANT GAMINE	Combination of OPPOSITES extra yang	Vertical + Petite
SOFT GAMINE	Combination of OPPOSITES extra yin	Curve + Petite

So, because we will be referring to them later when we start creating outfits and putting it all together, go ahead and record each of your definitions below. ONLY USE THE THREE CATEGORIES EXACTLY AS THEY ARE LAID OUT ABOVE. DO NOT ADD OR SUBTRACT OR SEPARATE ANYTHING. ALL THREE CATEGORIES GO TOGETHER.

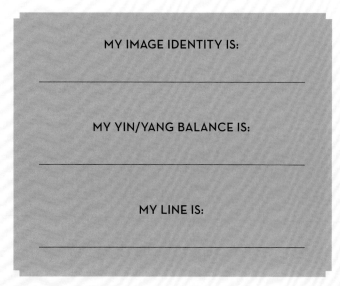

MY IMAGE IDENTITY IS:

_____

MY YIN/YANG BALANCE IS:

_____

MY LINE IS:

_____

CELEBRATION!!!! YOUR IMAGE IDENTITY IS HERE!!!!!!!

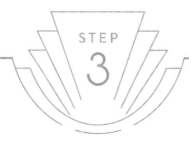

STEP 3

THE TRANSFORMATIONS

I am delighted to present to you the REVEALS of our ten beautiful friends, each a specific example of her IMAGE IDENTITY.

To help you view them and understand how they fit into the process, consider each as an INDIVIDUAL REPRESENTATIVE of her respective Image Identity. These photos are expressly presented to give you *the overall effect of the specific person*.

Don't try to decipher the separate elements of the technique here. (Later, we will delve deeper into how both Personal Line and the Color Seasons are expressed with visual illustrations and aids.)

I also highly recommend you don't look to see whom you identify with. *You are your own unique variety of whatever Image Identity you will be discovering as you reach that point of our journey.*

Instead, look to see how the individual qualities of each woman is focused. (I've given information on who each one is and what we did with her to help you see her in this manner. I've also included the height of each woman so you can have a clearer idea of how she appears in real life.)

Each of these women generously volunteered their time and energy. They are, each and every one, incredible and divine creatures! None are professional models. We simply tried to find unique and diverse women who we knew could showcase everything you are experiencing on our journey.

Each woman was asked to come in an outfit that she wears every day and wear her hair in her everyday way for her before shots. We did not manipulate anything in any way.

For their before picture, we did nothing except photograph them without makeup in their regular clothes. This is exactly how they all go about their daily affairs.

For their after shots, we of course styled them completely. There is no retouching of any kind—no filters, no Photoshopping, etc. Their afters are simply the results of applying my techniques head to toe!

You will see backgrounds that range from Caucasian to African-American, Latin, Asian, and East Indian, and sizes from XS to plus.

Their age range is equally diverse, from age sixteen to age eighty!

As you flip through the photos, remember, THESE ARE NOT MAKEOVERS!

I am opposed to the very concept of a "makeover." It runs counter to everything I believe in. No one needs to be *made over*. One of the first tenets we learned in this book is that YOU ARE EXACTLY WHO YOU ARE "SUPPOSED" TO BE!

Makeovers are someone else's vision superimposed on top of a person. They come from outside the person and are a façade that may or may not reflect anything about who the actual person underneath may be.

Instead, it is more accurate to view these as TRANSFORMATIONS. This is why we call them REVEALS. They come from defining the person's unique characteristics and then focusing these via my techniques. That is, in essence, exactly the opposite of what a makeover is based upon.

Each of our dazzling transformations reveals the INTEGRATION OF INNER AND OUTER that is each woman's unique STAR QUALITY—focused, polished, and refined. The spirit of each woman is the most exciting (and helpful) quality to look for and learn from.

YOU ARE EXACTLY WHO YOU ARE "SUPPOSED" TO BE!

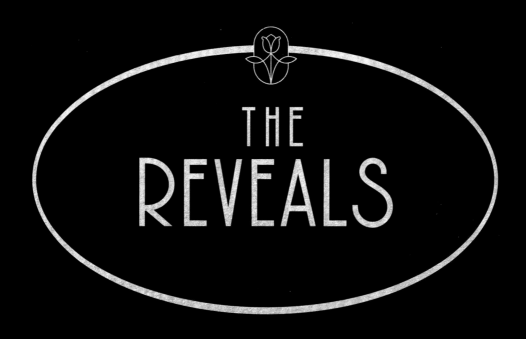

THE
REVEALS

YIN/YANG BALANCE: **YIN,**
with a yang undercurrent
HEIGHT: **5'5"**

Melissa was working as a nanny when she appeared to us like magic! She has the sweetest spirit and has a luminescence that the camera captures perfectly! After the shoot, she said perhaps she might do a bit of acting again. (We certainly hope so!)

In her reveal photo, you can see a great example of the silhouette of today that combines both body and clothes. Her dress is a stretch knit, what is often termed "body-con." This works in harmony with her shapely figure, highlighting it but not squeezing her into it. It's sensual but not overt. Simple often trumps in-your-face. This is the ideal example of the dress highlighting the woman, not the other way around!

THE COLOR: Carnation pink.
HAIR COLOR: We lightened her natural ash blond into a light cool blond.
HAIRSTYLE: A retro smooth glamour style with a peekaboo face frame.
MAKEUP: Soft pink/fuchsia.

Note her accessories are sparkly, which makes this more *casual evening*. They could also be simpler to take this dress into *fun daytime*.

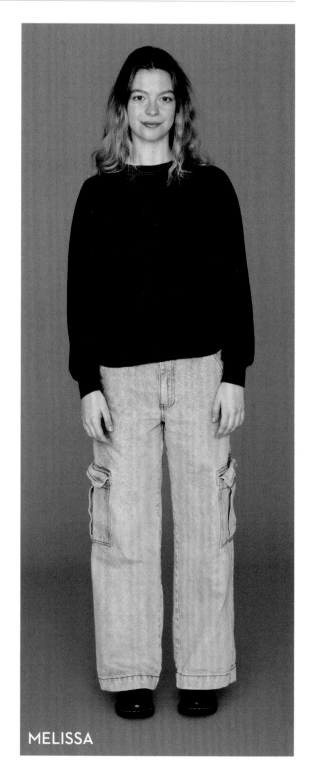

MELISSA

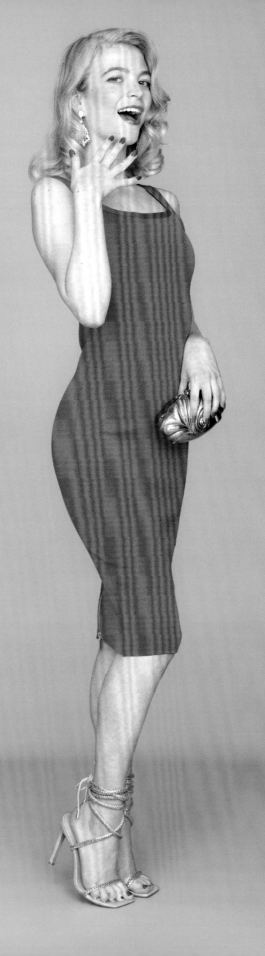

FLAMBOYANT GAMINE / VIVID WINTER

YIN/YANG BALANCE: **COMBINATION OF OPPOSITES**, extra yang
HEIGHT: 5'3"

We knew Zyana as the radiant hostess of a neighborhood restaurant. She had just completed her training in musical theater at an elite New York academy. Her real-life zest and buoyancy are perfectly captured by her photo!

In her reveal, you can see the juxtaposition of different colors, fabrics, and print forces your eye to travel in a broken, staccato line. The jacket is a wool blend, the skirt is ruffled, and the bralette is lace! Combined with the extra detail in accessories which use different materials ranging from enamel to pearl, you see how the *combination of opposites* manifests. At the same time, there is a definite color "pull-through" that connects all the disparate elements. Note particularly the elongated oval in the fuchsia earring, made of a combination of enamel, metal, and sparkle. It is oversized and both hangs on the ear and extends below. The shoes and bag are also important mixtures of texture and color. Black, hot pink, clear stones, and pearls. Shapes embody the combination of opposites that are geometric, a mixture of quirky and sophisticated!

THE COLORS: Various shades of shocking pink, deep cerise, and black.
HAIR COLOR: She had added some red tones to her hair, which, since she's a Vivid Winter, washed her out a bit. We reversed and slightly deepened it to a natural black.
HAIRSTYLE: We used her natural texture and then cut it into an asymmetrical shape.
MAKEUP: Deep smoky purples and vivid berry with pink.

Her outfit is a wonderful combo for anytime!

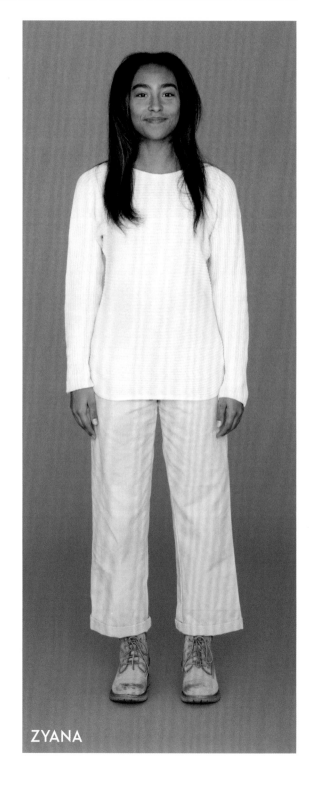

ZYANA

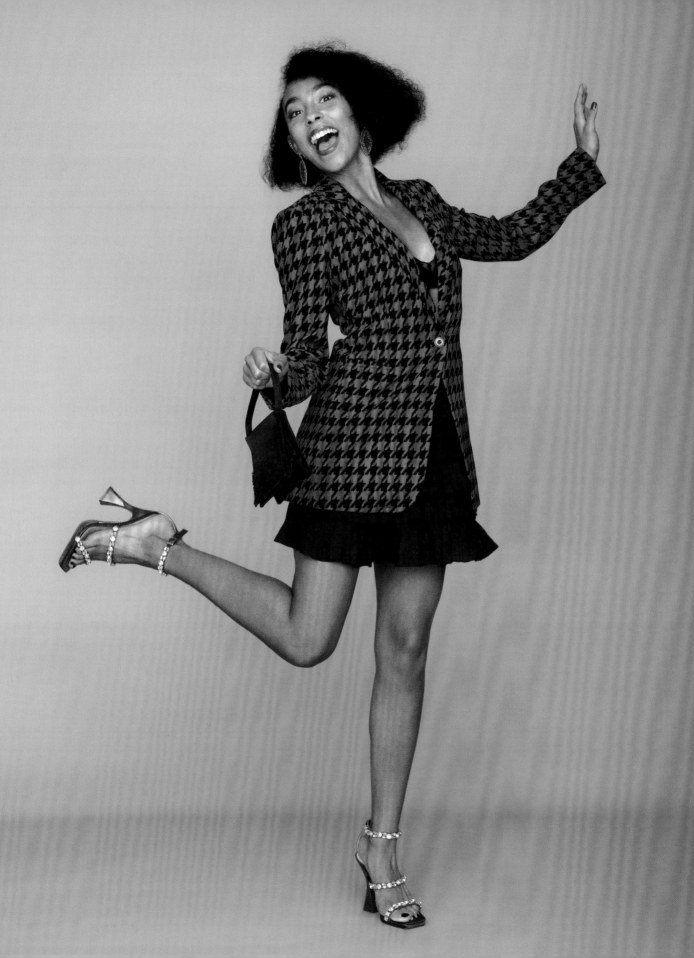

SOFT DRAMATIC / BRIGHT WINTER

YIN/YANG BALANCE: YANG,
with a pronounced yin undercurrent
HEIGHT: 5'9"

Rachael was the manager of a restaurant when we first encountered her. It's hard to capture all the facets of her. She was lovely in both manner and spirit and always had a brilliant smile for everyone she encountered. At the same time, you knew she had everything in total control. I always knew that there was a statuesque beauty just ready to bust out and dazzle, as you can easily see in her reveal!

I wanted Rachael to shine in something simple that would showcase her striking stature. We chose an elegant short silk dress in a monochromatic color scheme. Notice the soft blouson of the bodice that flows directly into the slim bottom of the dress. One long draped line that gracefully encompasses her divine figure.

THE COLOR: An icy lavender with black accessories. Simple, but with drama in shape.
HAIR COLOR: We kept her natural glossy black. (Why mess with perfection!)
HAIRSTYLE: We did a blunt cut with a smooth wave, keeping the overall length and with the front swept up and over to the side. Dramatic yet sophisticated.
MAKEUP: Soft smoky purple/pink eyes and frosted glossy fuchsia lips.

In her reveal, she is styled for an upscale nighttime or elegant daytime.

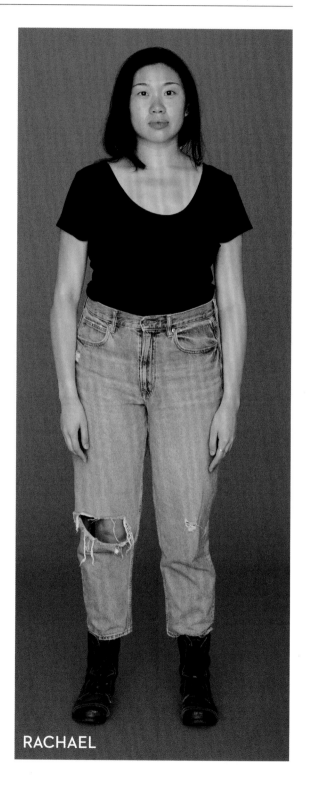

RACHAEL

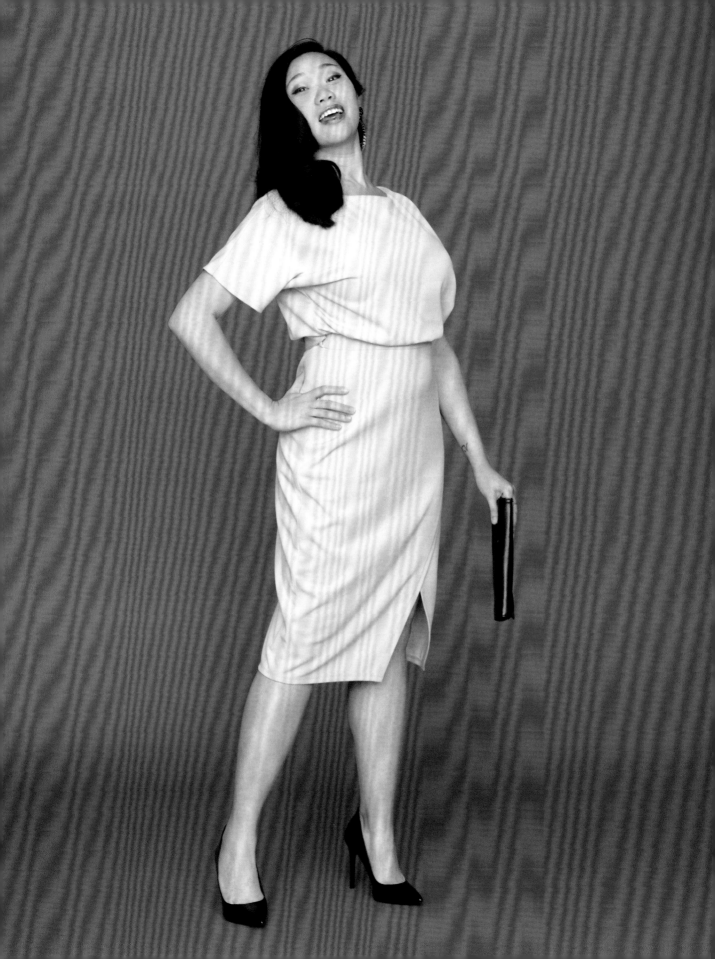

DRAMATIC CLASSIC / BRIGHT WINTER

BALANCED,
with a yang influence
HEIGHT: 5'1"

Rivka is an associate at a powerful New York agency. I knew under the surface lurked a powerhouse-in-waiting! She just needed a bit of encouragement and focus to bring this to life.

 Her natural balance called for simplicity yet a bit of structure with a tailored edge. Her coloring cried out for a dynamic combination. This is a riff on a tuxedo with menswear, but the fabric (with stretch) is totally another example of the body and fabric meshing to create a contemporary silhouette.

THE COLORS: A dramatic combo of jet and kelly. An all-black jacket/trouser suit with a kelly green knit shell. Then lapels and pockets in satin (again in kelly) create the striking effect. What you can't see due to her spirited pose is the same green satin piping on the side of the pants! Wowza!

 Her accessories are, again, simple and tailored. A clear cube on the ear, and patent leather platform pumps. (Notice the geometric-shape *pull-through*.)

HAIR COLOR: We kept her natural black. (Of course!)

HAIRSTYLE: Since she has an abundance of fabulous curl, we only wanted to get rid of the layers (which create straggly ends) and give it a blunt shape. Then we formed the waves a bit, sweeping it to one side and off her face. Form, but utilizing her natural texture.

MAKEUP: Red lips with smoky navy eyes focus the beauty of her pale skin/dark-hair/eyes contrast, while also effortlessly balancing and blending with the deep intensity of the clothing colors.

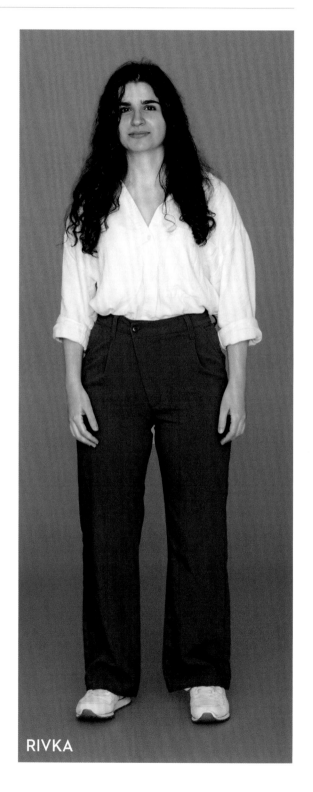

RIVKA

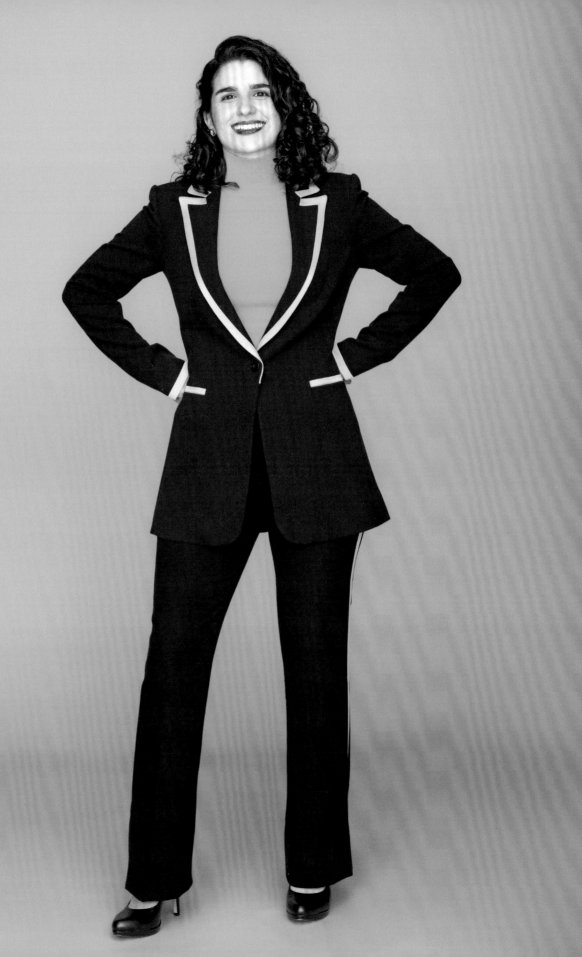

ROMANTIC / BRIGHT SPRING

YIN/YANG BALANCE: YIN, extreme (soft)
HEIGHT: 5'2¾"

Brianna was another magical creature that heaven seemed to send us. One day, when we were in a bit of a quandary searching for a Romantic who wasn't forthcoming, Brianna suddenly emerged behind a bar in our neighborhood eatery. She was in and out of town on tour (as actresses often are), so we hadn't realized this gem was right under our noses!

Her reveal is the most perfect expression of the inner and outer spirit of this talented lady! Encased in the delicate silk dress with the flowers and tiers, she really does seem like she is in an enchanted garden from another time! The thing that is striking is how the physical manifests when the clothes are in harmony with the person.

THE COLORS: A vibrant mixture of sunny yellows, peaches, and corals.
HAIR COLOR: We added warm lights to brighten her warm blonde.
HAIRSTYLE: A simple blunt shaping along a curved line and then a total set to frame her face in glorious curls.
MAKEUP: Warm shades of peach and soft golden tones highlight her glowing ivory complexion.

Look closely and you will see her shoes are delicate and accented with pearls. What you can't see underneath her voluminous curls are earrings in ivory with a hint of peach.

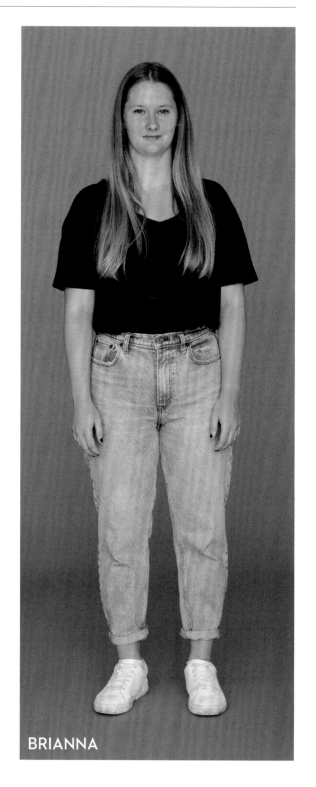

BRIANNA

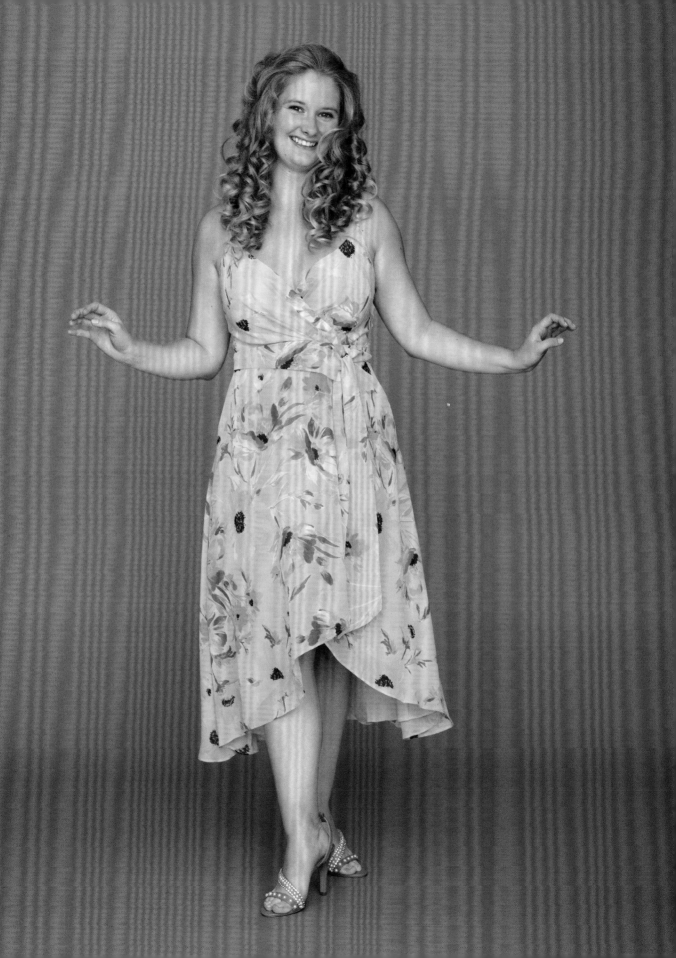

FLAMBOYANT NATURAL / VIVID WINTER

YIN/YANG BALANCE: YANG, bold, blunt
HEIGHT: 5'6"

Serena is a combination of seraph and student! This amazing teenager was busy manning an upscale jewelry boutique when we found her. Not only that, during our photo shoot, while on the sidelines, she was also studying for her SATs! We really felt like the goddesses were working for us with these wonderful gals, and Serena might actually be one of the angels who dropped into our life!

What was important to us was to combine the free spirit and high style of the Flamboyant Natural with Serena's youth. We emphasized the light-hearted combo of a jacket with miniskirt that is a *bit of a suit but not really*! Combined with a cropped top that is a bold horizontal stripe, and you have something that only a fresh young beauty could rock! Then, of course, there are the boots!!

THE COLORS: It's all about the freshness of the sapphire blue and pure white while at the same time focusing on her vivid contrast. Drama and freshness are the two key elements. There are two color pull-throughs, the obvious blue, but also the white in the crop top and boots.

HAIR COLOR: We kept her deep cool brunette.

HAIRSTYLE: A bit of blunt cutting to keep a strong shape and allow maximum volume. Then just a release of her wild and wonderful curls.

MAKEUP: Keeping her cool vivid palette of red lips and navy eyes. We also wanted it to be simple, so her beaming smile is the focus of her face!

The accent on youthful fun meant we wanted to capitalize on the sixties nod with both the boots (not necessarily made for walkin'!), but also, if you look closely at her earrings, you'll notice triple hanging balls adding that touch of pop on the ear!

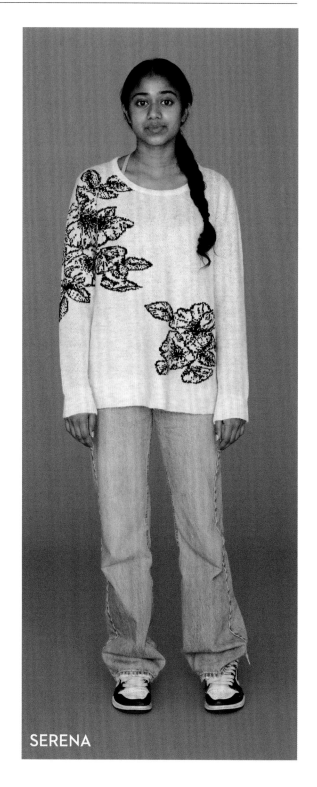

SERENA

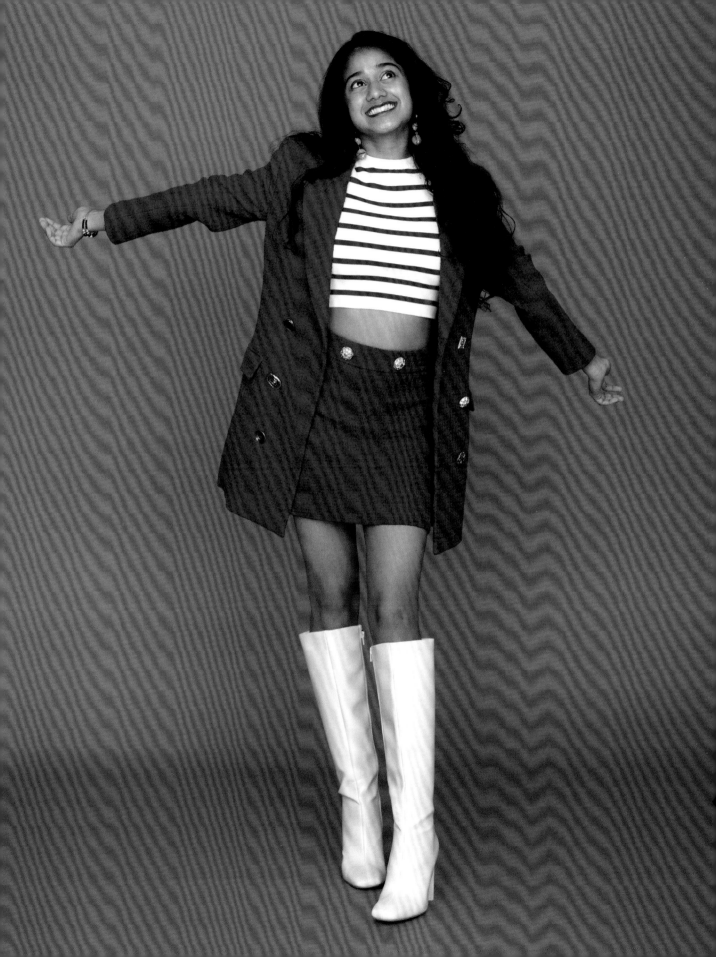

SOFT CLASSIC / VIVID SUMMER

YIN/YANG BALANCE: BALANCED, with a yin influence
HEIGHT: 5'4"

Our discovery of Margaret was a combination of serendipity and divine intervention. Susan and I were guests at an anniversary celebration of a beloved neighborhood trattoria when out of the blue, this lovely lady appeared with her partner. I knew, in an instant, we had found our Soft Classic!

Having emigrated from Poland many decades ago, Margaret had raised her children (now fully grown) and become a successful real estate mogul. Not only that, turns out she lived very close to us and was "hiding in plain sight" all along.

We knew it was all about realizing her refined elegance while keeping a bit of wit front and center. The answer was a nod to the fifties but totally "today" that this riff on a Dior New Look design suggests. The full skirt, yet very fitted, captures that vintage haute feeling. On the other hand, the fabric of a crushed metallic brocade, along with the three-quarter sleeves, the sheer net of the skirt's inlay, and the open tailored collar, keeps things rooted in the present day.

Notice the combination of classic, timeless refinement in the choice of accessories, yet always with a twist that is strictly millennial. Especially fun are her elegant d'Orsay pumps with the very oversized bows and naughtily wacky heel.

THE COLORS: Elegant champagne and cream, with a dusting of metallic rose gold. Pearls and shimmer add the final touches.
HAIR COLOR: We updated her color with refined, face-framing highlights of cool blonde.
HAIRSTYLE: We evened out the layers for a smoother cut and then created a modern updo, with very specific large curls on top that give this queen her crown of glory.

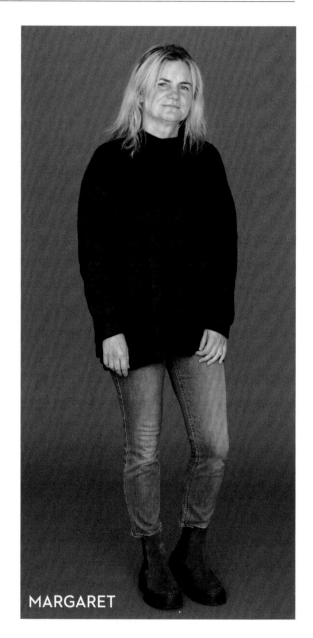

MARGARET

MAKEUP: Dusty plums and mauve eyes with soft rose lips and cheeks.

The result—haute elegance while being just a bit irreverent—creates a feeling of offhand glamour we are thrilled to offer up as Margaret's reveal.

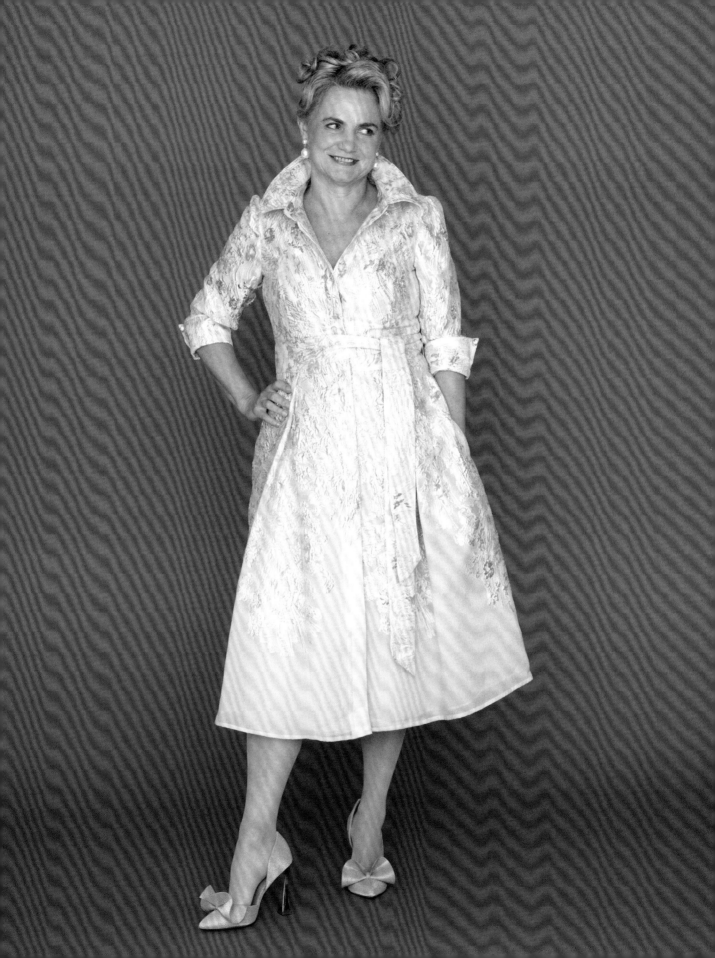

SOFT NATURAL / VIVID AUTUMN

YIN/YANG BALANCE: YANG, with a yin undercurrent
HEIGHT: 5'3"

I knew I wanted Paige to be in the book when I first was enraptured by her radiant smile. Paige is a *personality-plus ball of fire*! She has the combination of a bit of sass with a lot of class that lights up any room she enters! She is an agent-in-training at a prestigious company that rules its domain.

Capturing her vivaciousness, her vibrant spirit, and her power while not sacrificing her fresh appeal was the goal. Also, the fire of her coloring adds zest and zip. So it was a no-brainer when we came up with this animal print, in a silk dress topped with a shrug! Everything is like a riff that says, "I've got it all, but I don't take it too seriously." It's all for fun but clearly thought out. Freely put together, while at the same time, definitely all planned out. This is a silhouette that incorporates a lot of skin in the overall effect.

THE COLORS: Hot yellow-gold and deep espresso.
HAIR COLOR: We kept her natural chestnut with a reddish tint that is emphasized by the colors of the outfit and makeup.
HAIRSTYLE: Full and voluminous while keeping it loose. A blunt cut on a curved outline, then formed in waves around the face. The rest is a cascade of her natural wave (which we simply gave a bit more shape).
MAKEUP: All bronze and copper, with a bit of frost here and there.

To finish this, we added a bit of golden shimmer to the accessories. It's in keeping with the sassy fun that is just a bit of unexpected gloss. Look closely and you'll notice extremely oversized hoops on her ears, a big chunk of gold bracelet, and then the purse of metallic gold fabric that is ready for a good swing!

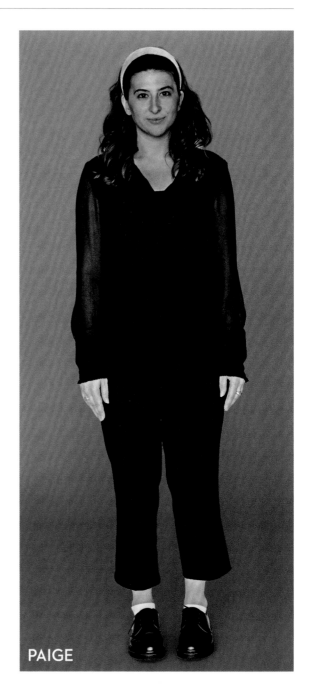

PAIGE

Shoes are nude but with crisscross straps going up her leg with the open front that showcases bronze polish on the toes!

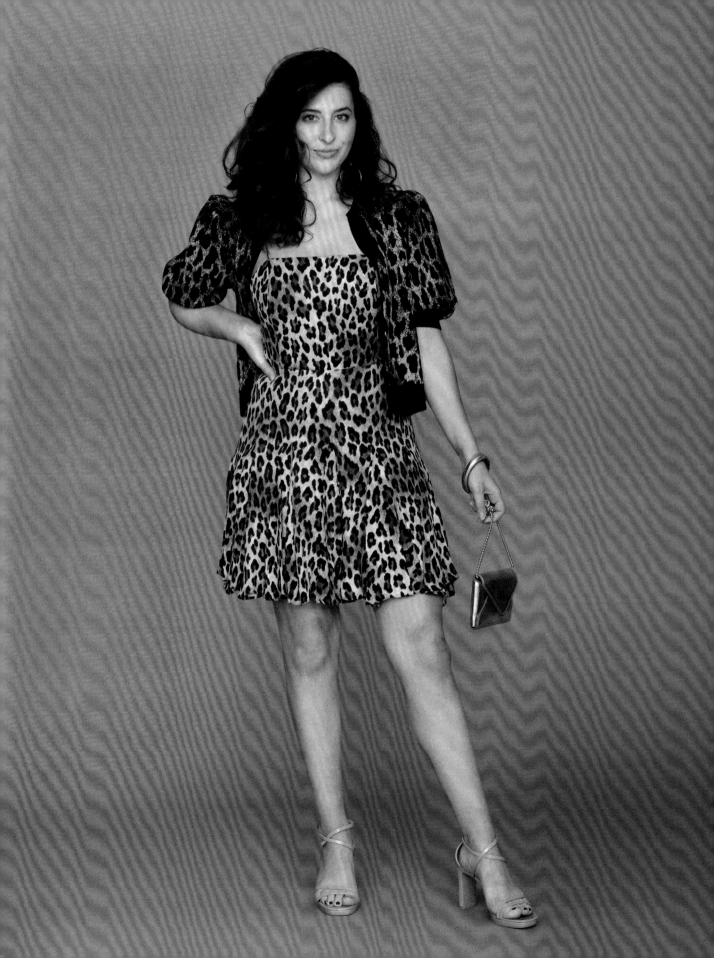

SOFT GAMINE / BRIGHT WINTER

YIN/YANG BALANCE: **COMBINATION OF OPPOSITES, extra Yin**

HEIGHT: 5'1"

What do I need to say about a young lady whose name has the perfect description of who she is as the first two syllables? She is a student but moonlights in a festive trattoria. Susan and I were charmed out of our skins at our very first encounter. When it came time to do the photos, there was no question we wanted to include this darling, if both she and her mother would be on board. Happily for us, we have the magical results to reveal.

Here again, her youth was very important to honor, but at the same time, we wanted to capture her budding sophistication. A playful dress with just a bit of flirt that harked back to the twenties was the answer here. Angelisa is an updated flapper ready to fly. There is both a sweetness and a sauciness to her dress, in the fabric, the silhouette, and the color combo. It's an embossed quilted texture that is totally surprising (just like her!). The best part of her style story is her on-camera demeanor. Actually quite shy and soft-spoken, we took the greatest joy in how she instantly became the life of the party as soon as she was in front of the camera. To top things off, right now Angelisa's future goal is to become a forensic detective. We know she will do whatever she sets her mind to.

THE COLORS: A combination of hot pink and cherry red woven together. (It's more about the effect of the combo than the separate colors. Very unexpected and very exuberant!)

HAIR COLOR: We kept her natural very dark cool brown color.

HAIRSTYLE: Keeping with the 1920s, we went for a blunt, chin-length bob (curved under), with eye-framing smooth bangs.

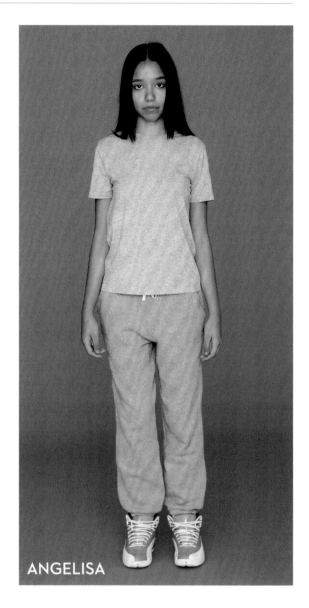

ANGELISA

MAKEUP: Fresh, in keeping with her youth, but rosy red with soft smoked-purple eyes.

Now, her accessories bear a close look. These are vital for her staccato line. Red flats with a tapered toe. A red fringed and beaded bag (pure twenties!). What you can barely see beneath her bob is a hanging cherry earring.

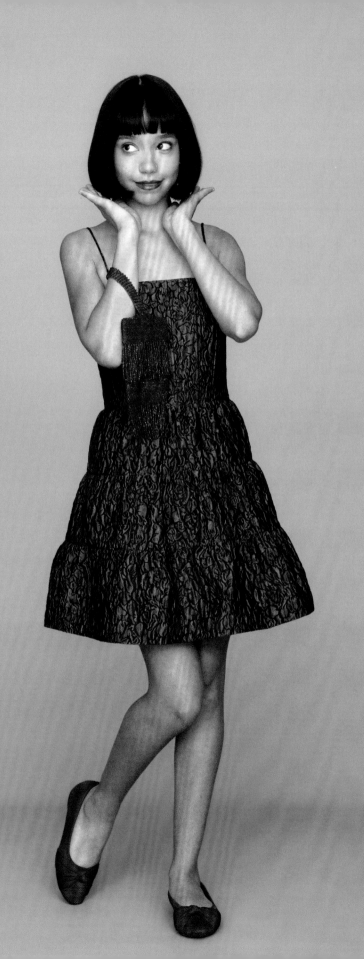

DRAMATIC / FIERY AUTUMN

YIN/YANG BALANCE: YANG, extreme (sharp)
HEIGHT: 5'8"

If you were to look up a synonym for Veronica online there should only be one: *dynamo!* Otherwise, it would take volumes to describe this one-of-kind beauty. She is the undisputed queen and organizer of her neighborhood. An opera singer and actress, if Sarah Bernhardt were alive, Veronica would surely be her number one rival. Yet she also has a quiet power and dignity that I wanted to capture.

My goal was pure Old Hollywood leading lady but in an updated manner. I wanted the luxury of all cream in fabrics that suggested the finest wool and cashmere. And of course, we needed a true ensemble effect, complete with scarf and coat. (If I could have found a Russian wolfhound to rent for the day, I definitely would have added it to her reveal!)

There is nothing to break the elegant mono color scheme of ivory/cream except for the dark brown buttons, which add just a hint of wit to this outfit. The wonderful thing about this reveal is that it whispers—never shouts—Veronica's stature. Along with the throwaway of the gorgeous coat, this reveal showcases her absolute confidence. Elegant, sophisticated, and always ready for her close-up!

THE COLORS: A monochrome scheme of all cream and ivory tells the entire story. But also, it's the luxury of the fabric that allows these colors to make such a powerful statement.

HAIR COLOR: We gave Veronica an overall color of rich auburn.

HAIRSTYLE: After a simple cut, we channeled a bit of forties with a hint of victory roll. It's a riff on a French twist in the back with the upsweep in front. Not a dead-on throwback but an updated version. Totally modern, but evocative of a Golden Age movie star.

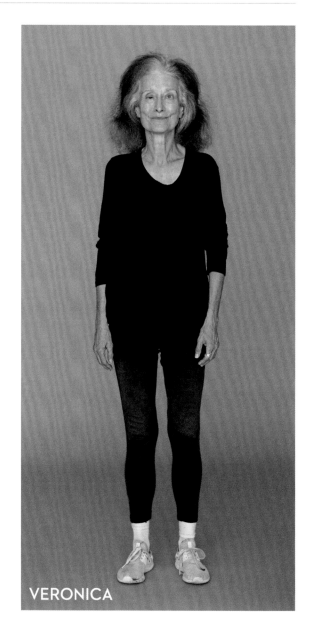

VERONICA

MAKEUP: Hints of tawny peach with gold and jade eyes.

Her accessories are simple, simple, simple. Merely a hunk of sculpted gold on the ear. The shoes are pale sand suede booties with just the tip showing.

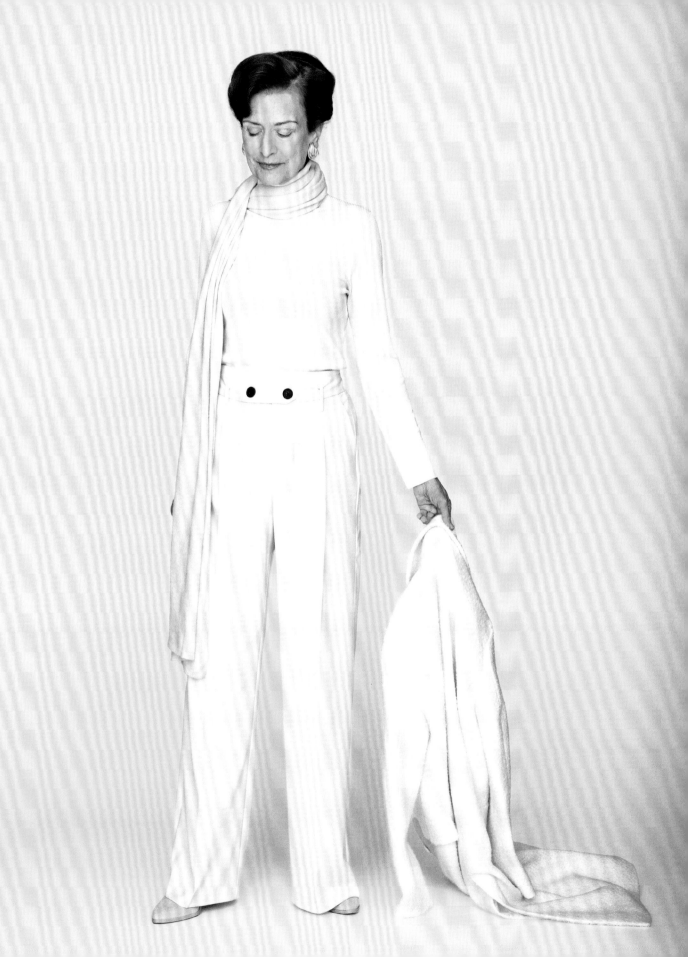

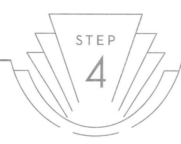

IMAGE IDENTITIES OVERHAULED

REFRESHED, REFURBISHED, RENOVATED PREAMBLE

Now that you have clarified your actual Image Identity, the question is: *What does this mean in this new environment we live in, and how can I help you maneuver through it?*

I'm in the field with clients every day. Nothing keeps me more updated than being confronted with the actual merchandise that is in the stores. Especially in today's world of fast fashion, with its dizzyingly rapid turnovers, you really can't hang on to any rigid ideas that might have been relevant in the past.

At the same time, the whole point of having personal style is to connect with the things that are timeless totems of your individual identity. Without those things that help communicate the core elements of who you are and what you are about on this planet, you have no chance of developing an authentic style.

Without these, you are just at the mercy of whatever crazy trend is being sold and is going to be passé by the next week! As I always say: "Today's trends are already yesterday's news!"

Yet, there is definitely a way to both stay a citizen of the modern world *and* keep your feet firmly planted in your own clear style standards. To do this, you have to navigate the difference between what is wonderful in today's clothes and what is simply passing fancy.

It really all boils down to staying true to what we have found to be your style foundation: *knowing how to accommodate your* PERSONAL LINE *in a complementary silhouette.* The more facile you get doing this simple thing, the more you will be able to be a STYLE STAR: always current, yet always true to yourself!

HARMONY IS HAPPENING

The very best of what has changed today from yesterday is the part of fashion that connects with our ever-evolving humanity. It's what I call the *symbiosis of our inner angels with the design of the times*!

The wonderful thing about today is the constant movement toward openness in our society. There is one word that best sums up what I see as the major connection point where both fashion and our human experience are united: FLEXIBILITY.

To me, the advent of the new silhouettes merges perfectly with the ideals of the more open acceptance of all the different facets of humanity our world is moving toward.

We live in a world that is far less rigid than in the past, and doesn't that amalgamate beautifully with all things regarding the new approach to silhouette we have been learning? Less rigidity, more flexibility!

What that means, however, is that we definitely need a different approach to delineating the specifics of each Image Identity than we had in the past. It can't be fixed and unbending. If society is more adaptable and clothes are more pliable, then we must also update the way you use your Image Identity to embrace this new FLEXIBILITY.

There can be no list of hard and fast "recs" (recommendations) for each image category. Such a list today would not be merely curating outdated fashions, it would be completely useless and totally irrelevant to the clothes that are wearable today.

LESS RIGIDITY, MORE FLEXIBILITY!

REMEMBER: CLOTHES DON'T HAVE IMAGE IDENTITIES, PEOPLE DO!

I realize it is tempting to wish for a simple inventory of details for each Identity. That is simply not possible today. Such a list would, by its very existence, be a false guide that would take you down a myriad of rabbit holes of misleading information. You would spin your wheels forever following these lists and still come home empty-handed!

First, you would never even find those types of clothes in the stores. They don't exist the same way they used to. Even if they did, you would find yourself forced into a rigid box that would totally clip your style wings! *There is no authenticity possible when you have been chained into a stereotyped box from the past!*

Today, even amidst an overload of some really bad fast fashion, there are fabulous designs and unlimited opportunities available. It would be verging on criminal if I didn't give you the way to avail yourself of all the possibilities you have at your disposal!

Style by algorithm is an oxymoron. There is no mathematical type of categorization that will not end up with you in a box. Style is personal. Lists are generic. And algorithms will keep you rooted in the past. An algorithm is based on what you've already done. Style is about harnessing potential!

Here's an example: I could come up with a fabulous two-piece pantsuit that had waist suppression in a stretch blend that I could fit beautifully on at least five women with different Image Identities. The silhouette would be different on each lady due to the way the fabric interacted with each body.

Now, if I were shopping by a list of recs, I might not find that this fits the specifics of anyone's list! The waist suppression alone would have eliminated it from anyone with Vertical on their recs! Yet, waist suppression in this fabric and cut wouldn't disrupt any bit of a Vertical.

This is exactly how the NEW SILHOUETTE works.

On the other hand, everyone cannot wear everything! That notion is not simply false, it's pretty ridiculous! What we want today is SPECIFICITY WITHOUT RIGIDITY!

THE NEW SILHOUETTE: YOUR TICKET TO FREEDOM!

PERSONALITY IS NOT IMAGE IDENTITY

The other thing to mention now is the difference in how you identify the inner part of your Image Identity. Since we are more fluid in the way we define clothes, we also need a more expansive approach to how we perceive and express the so-called *essence* part of your style. A method that allows the full extent of *who you are on the inside* to come out, without sticking you with a label that is less complete than you are!

What I'm getting at here is that the part of Image Identity that used to be defined as your inner self also has got to be redefined in a broader way.

Today, with fluidity as our goal, we don't want to categorize your inner self. It's not the way to express your soul. If we were to assign personality traits, essences, and the like, we would, again, just be putting you in a box. *A soul box is just as limiting as a clothing box.*

Whether you want to refer to your inner self as personality or essence, the only way to truly capture your spirit is to recognize it as ephemeral. To realize that trying to put it into any fixed category is tantamount to catching soap bubbles and stuffing them in a jar!

It is never one thing. We always are growing, changing, and evolving. That is built into our DNA. Life moves forward. So do we. Our personality is totally dependent on SITUATION. It is not fixed. Nor is it what others perceive.

You have a multitude of inner qualities. You don't want them stifled by a one-note approach to how they are communicated in your appearance. Therefore, we also need to reflect this in how we define your Image Identity.

I want to move you away from the older idea that your Image Identity is one thing. Instead of categorizing your inner qualities, I want you to learn to *express them.*

Your inner self is going to emerge on its own. You don't need to clarify it as a goal. It happens naturally as a *result*. The *flavor* of you is inherent. It flows out automatically by being specific in the choices you make.

You will find that the most specific way to capture your individual qualities today is through Situation and Intent. This will be done through the actual choices you make in creating outfits. I will give you clear techniques to do just that when we get into the sections where we shop, and where we *put it all together*.

But let's not worry about that right now. At this point, think of this as simply the preface to introduce the new way of defining each IMAGE IDENTITY.

These are the core elements of each Image Identity updated for today's world. The purpose they serve is to help you Enhance, Clarify, and Focus. My goal here is to help you distill the basics of your Image Identity that are the requirements needed to use this technique.

Here's a tip: Requirements are not rules. All art has requirements in order to communicate clearly. Without them, you just have hodgepodge. Music without any structure is just noise.

Rules, on the other hand, do not allow for individual expression. They are the *opposite* of requirements.

These guidelines are absolutely NOT rules. *Think of them as tickets to your freedom.* They are simple, easy, and direct. Without them as your basis, you cannot harness the power of your style.

Remember that your Image Identity is not meant to put you in a box. Exactly the opposite! As we've discussed, everyone is made up of a multitude of qualities.

But if you want your STYLE MESSAGE to be communicated clearly, it requires CLARITY in order to achieve FOCUS. Nothing will defeat your style more quickly and completely than sending out MIXED MESSAGES.

Now, on the other hand, Image Identity is NOT the same as your personal aesthetic. That, like the aforementioned personality/essence, is not something that can be quantified. It is movable, not fixed.

Our personal aesthetics evolve over our life. For instance, I'm sure there are foods you disdained as a child but in time learned to love.

For myself, up until my twenties, the very mention of avocado turned my stomach. Truly, I had such an aversion to the thought of that mushy green abomination, it was beyond the pale. Also, I was positive this was a permanent position of mine!

Well, boy, was I surprised when one weekend I was a houseguest at a friend's summer cottage, and she served an avocado dish for lunch. Starving, and with no other choice (being the polite Midwestern boy I was trained to be), I bit the bullet and prepared to endure one giant yuckadoo!

Holy guacamole! I loved this! Hmm, good lesson for me. Never say never!

The point is, while it's fulfilling and important to know what our taste is, at the same time, it's important to remember that our proclivities evolve as we evolve. The moral is: *Don't be too adamant about what your current aesthetic is.* It can, and will, change with time. It's always acceptable, while at the same time, it always can be better.

On the other hand, your Image Identity does not limit your expression. It is a VEHICLE. One of the big misinterpretations of my work is the conflation of Image Identity with a certain look.

A "look" is not your STYLE. You can have as many looks as your taste, creativity, and skill allow. This is not a reflection or indication of your Image Identity. As I've said before, your Image Identity is NOT a type. It's also not a look.

I like to describe it as your STYLE COUNTRY. Within each "country" there are unlimited places where your style can reside. *It's the language you use to communicate your style.* The story you use this language to create is based on the specific time, place, and situation you find yourself in and want to convey.

THE ICONS AND OLD HOLLYWOOD

IT'S THE ARTISTRY AND THE FOCUS

> *Don't let's ask for the moon, we have the stars.*
> —*NOW, VOYAGER*

Now, let's also take a moment to discuss the ICONs for each Image Identity, the how and why they come from OLD HOLLYWOOD.

The first thing to remember about the Icons is that they are representatives of how FOCUS is the technical goal for all your efforts.

When things are cohesive, *you get the definition of* character, situation, purpose, *and everything that*

helps you send your own personal STAR QUALITY *out to the world!*

So, the one place we can turn to for examples of how this works is the OLD HOLLYWOOD STUDIO SYSTEM. There are elements of this setup that are crucial to our work and simply cannot exist in the system that creates the celebrities of today.

(This is not to say there is nothing relevant about

style in today's celebrity culture, but it has a very different makeup, in terms of both purpose and what it expresses. Later on we will go into today's celebrity culture, but that is a very different landscape.)

In the days of the studio system, the first thing they did with a new actress was put her through the star factory. Each studio had its own version of this, which combined the world's greatest artists in design, hair, makeup, lighting, and coaching. Their goal was to discover/identify and then create the indelible image of this newcomer. Everything about her image was created and concocted to clarify her as a one-of-a-kind supernova—a Jean Harlow, a Joan Crawford, etc. They needed to be *the one and only,* and this is how they created that persona.

You have to remember that at this point, the movies were star driven. It was the stars that drove audiences to the theaters. So it was in the studios' best financial interest to develop the actors into the audience magnets that filled their seats! (They also owned the theaters until the Supreme Court put an end to that in a landmark 1948 ruling, which was the beginning of the end of the old studio system.)

It's this development of stars that we are looking to borrow techniques from. There is nothing like that today. In those days, the studios' control of the image of each performer meant that *specificity* was key. Every aspect of their image was honed and focused.

Today, without the studios behind them, there is an entirely different structure for how artists are presented. While they have celebrity stylists, they are also promoting specific designers with endorsement deals. In short, today the focus is less about the actress and more about the clothes.

This is not to say that some of the clothes are not fabulous, because they are. Also, some of the cos-

tume designers for the individual films of today are extraordinary. Sandy Powell could easily give Edith Head a run for her money! (Both are, and were, absolute geniuses at their art, as were, and are, many other amazing designers.)

Now, of course, there were many problems with the Old Hollywood studio system. The hyper-control that kept actors in a version of indentured servitude, for one. Then there was the really indefensible lack of representation. (More is coming on that later, including updates and exemplars.)

Also, there is the fact that we are living in another era! While there are clothes that can translate directly from those films (see either of the Hepburns' outfits, for instance), as we have previously discussed, there has been a sea change of possibilities that exist today that were not available at that earlier time.

The other thing to remember is how we define the term "ICON."

In style terms, an Icon *must withstand the passage of time*. This requires both the indelible style that is timeless, as well as the *vehicle* that allows her to continue to be known well past her initial fame.

There are definitely prominent celebrities around who may achieve this status. But our media today is fickle. It doesn't, as a rule, provide the platform that is lasting. Time will tell, of course, but for us at this time, we have the advantage of the artistry of those "star-making" factories, along with the lasting imagery these classic films provide.

I want to stress again, it's the artistry of the FOCUS we are looking for in using these Icons as symbols. They are NOT role models to imitate. Imitation is never the goal in style. Learning what has created their successful timelessness is what we need to mine and utilize.

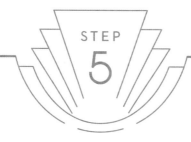

STEP
5

IN A NUTSHELL

THE CORE OF EACH IMAGE IDENTITY
DEFINED AND ILLUSTRATED

Now, you will see in your individual Image Identity breakdowns below that there is listed, first, the ICON. This is a timeless example of a star created by the studio star factory who is the clearest example of your Image Identity. Her image has the specific focus that has been honed and clarified. Her clothes and appearance elements have the FOCUS that you can learn from. (And again, I'm not asking you to necessarily identify with her. She is simply the epitome of the technique expressed, which you can learn from.)

What I've also done is give EXEMPLARS: women from that same era who did not get the prominence they deserved. These women may not have the same clarity in the image that was presented, but they are examples of their respective Image Identities just the same. (Some of these you may not be as familiar with as the Icons, but you can easily find numerous photos and descriptions of them through an online search.) These women come from all backgrounds. They each have a body of work that, through its excellence, allows them the status of timelessness.

You will also see three illustrations of possible

Head-To-Toes (HTTs) for each Image Identity. The first is an updated iconic version, the second is a creative version, and the third is an illustration of a plus-size translation. Each one also is painted to show examples of color, hair, and makeup for the specific HTT.

There is a caption under each to help you visualize the illustration in real life (including proportions). These include height, seasonal color designation, and fabric of outfit.

Remember not to look at these as "I would or would not wear this outfit." They all illustrate POSSIBILITIES. Ultimately, your choices will be determined by your own personal needs regarding your life's situations.

Also, refrain from focusing on your perception of the body and trying to compare it to what you believe yours looks like. IT'S SOLELY ABOUT THE CLOTHING. Your learning will come from seeing the way Personal Line translates into Silhouette in each of these specific renderings.

THIS IS PLAYTIME

Remember something very important: This is supposed to be FUN. Be clear, be specific, stay focused on cohesiveness, but also PLAY. Style is delightful. This is not school. There are no tests and there are no "fashion police" involved. This is simply acquiring the TECHNIQUE that will let you fly!

Note: Remember, your IMAGE IDENTITY is determined by the combination of, first, your YIN/ YANG BALANCE, and, second, your PERSONAL LINE. These three components always go together this way. There are no additions, subtractions, or exceptions. If this isn't what you've determined for yourself at this time, you've come to incorrect conclusions. This means you need to go back and rework the relevant section and replay its games until you have these aligned.

STYLE IS DELIGHTFUL— THIS IS PLAYTIME!

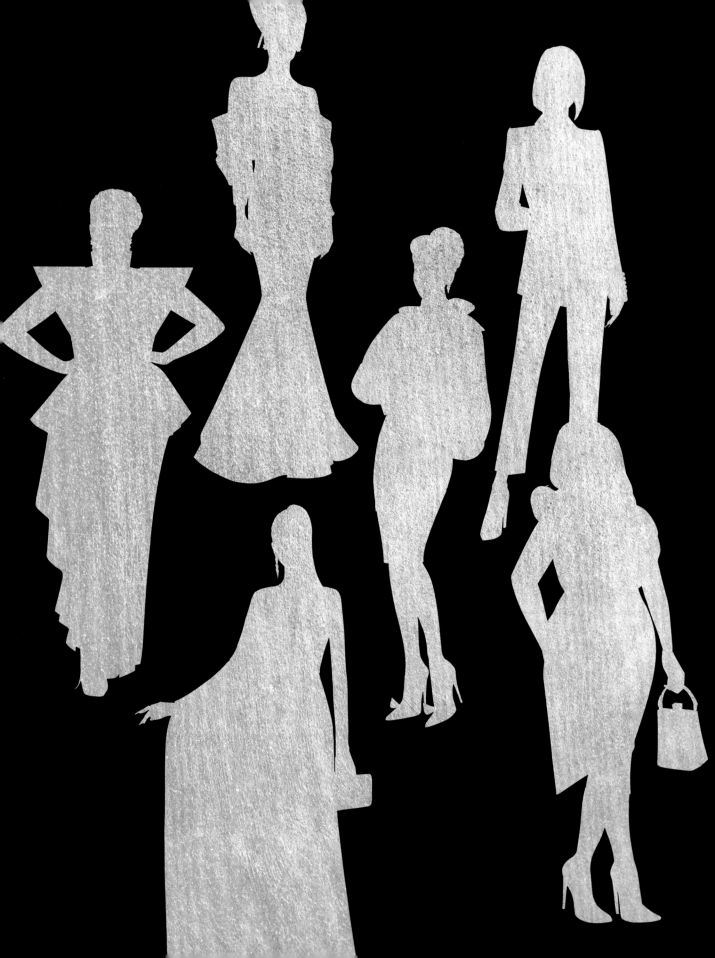

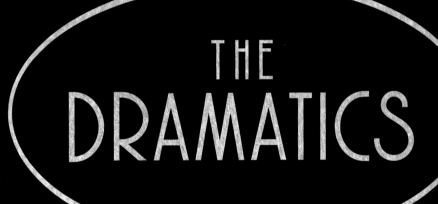

THE
DRAMATICS

DRAMATIC

THE DECO DYNAMO

YIN/YANG BALANCE: YANG, extreme (sharp)

LINE: VERTICAL + NARROW (any height is possible but usually five foot six and over)

SILHOUETTE: You always want an outline that is sleek and narrow. When looking at it, the eye needs to travel straight down in one unbroken vertical. It can be tailored with more structure, or it can be flowing, as long as it flows *down* instead of *out*.

ICON: Katharine Hepburn

EXEMPLARS: Diahann Carroll, Anna May Wong, Katy Jurado, France Nuyen

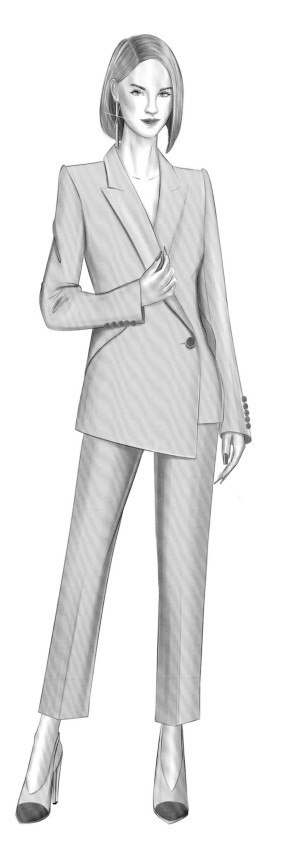

UPDATED ICONIC

Height: 5'6"
Season: Gentle Spring
Fabric: Fine twill

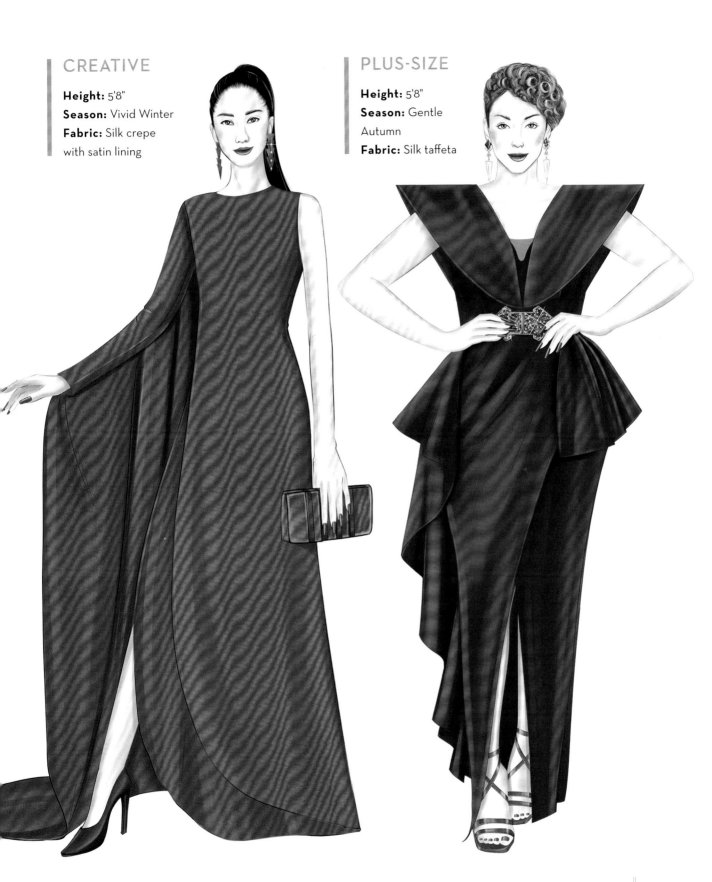

CREATIVE

Height: 5'8"
Season: Vivid Winter
Fabric: Silk crepe
with satin lining

PLUS-SIZE

Height: 5'8"
Season: Gentle
Autumn
Fabric: Silk taffeta

SOFT DRAMATIC

THE DIVA

YIN/YANG BALANCE: YANG, with a pronounced yin undercurrent

LINE: VERTICAL+ CURVE (any height is possible, but usually five foot six and over)

SILHOUETTE: You need both a strong vertical (long, unbroken) along with a soft, curved or draped outline. When one is looking at you, the eye needs to travel in one unbroken vertical downward but should also have curve or drape, especially on top. If there is flow, it still needs to be elongated.

ICON: Sophia Loren

EXEMPLARS: Lena Horne, Sara Montiel, Saloma, Shohreh Aghdashloo

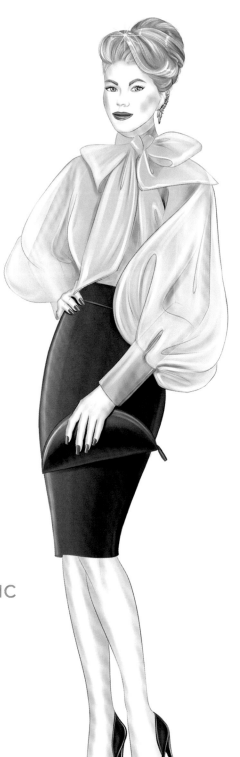

UPDATED ICONIC

Height: 5'7"
Season: Dusty Summer
Fabric: Organza blouse, stretch gabardine skirt

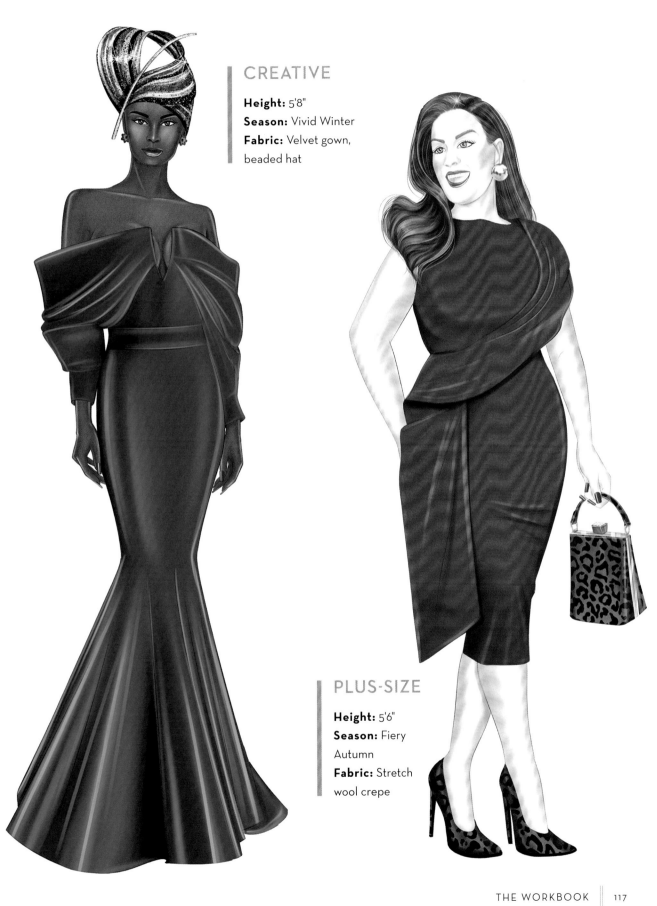

CREATIVE

Height: 5'8"
Season: Vivid Winter
Fabric: Velvet gown,
beaded hat

PLUS-SIZE

Height: 5'6"
Season: Fiery
Autumn
Fabric: Stretch
wool crepe

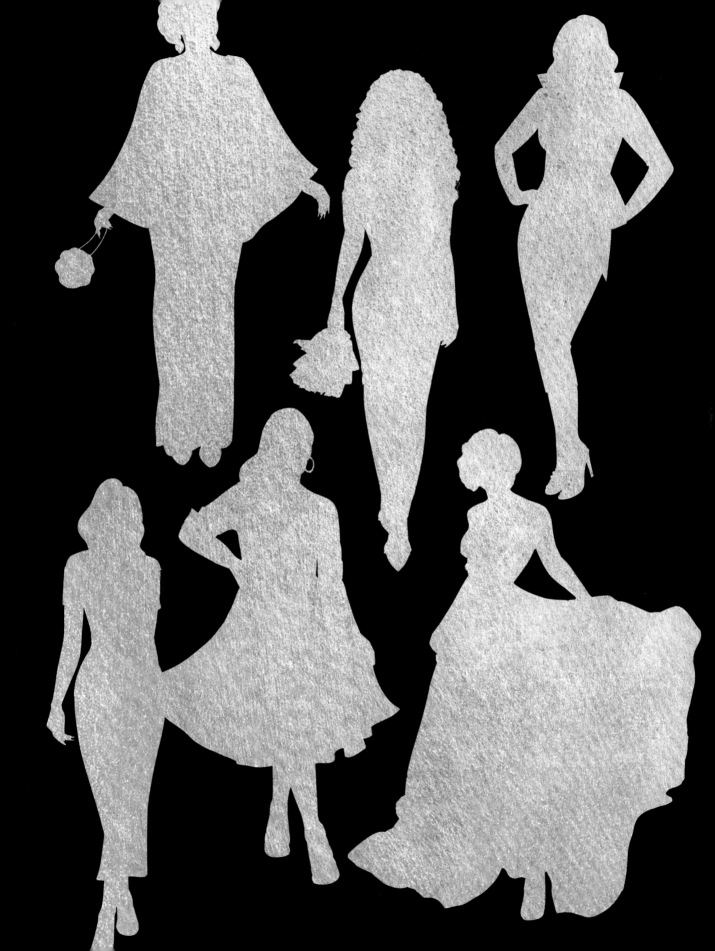

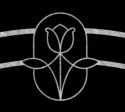

THE
ROMANTICS

ROMANTIC

LA BELLE

YIN/YANG BALANCE: YIN, extreme (soft)

LINE: CURVE + DOUBLE CURVE (height: under five foot six)

SILHOUETTE: You need an outline that is soft, allowing the curves to be accommodated. When one is looking at you, the eye needs to travel around both curves. It can either skim the body (not too tight) or flow outward. Fluidity is important. Nothing stiff.

ICON: Marilyn Monroe

EXEMPLARS: Etta James, Rekha, Lotus Long, Renee Torres

UPDATED ICONIC

Height: 5'4"
Season: Soft Summer
Fabric: Silk chiffon

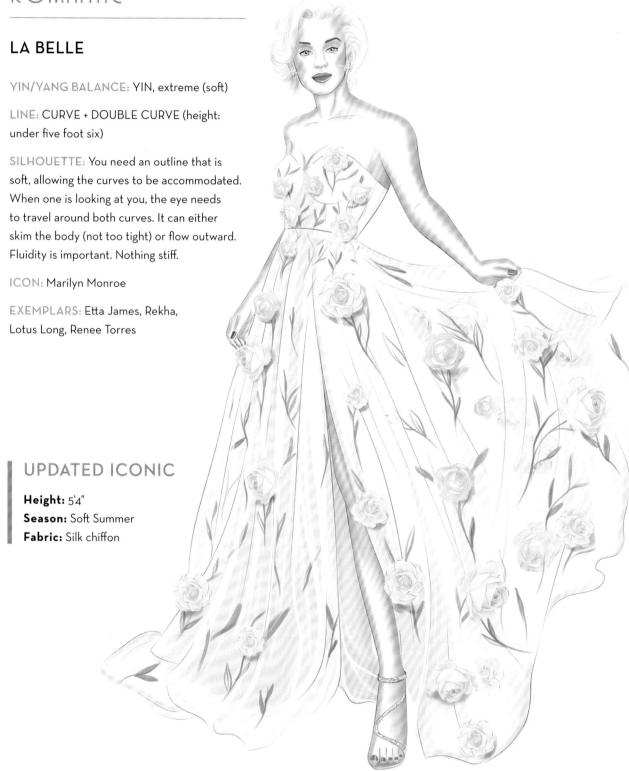

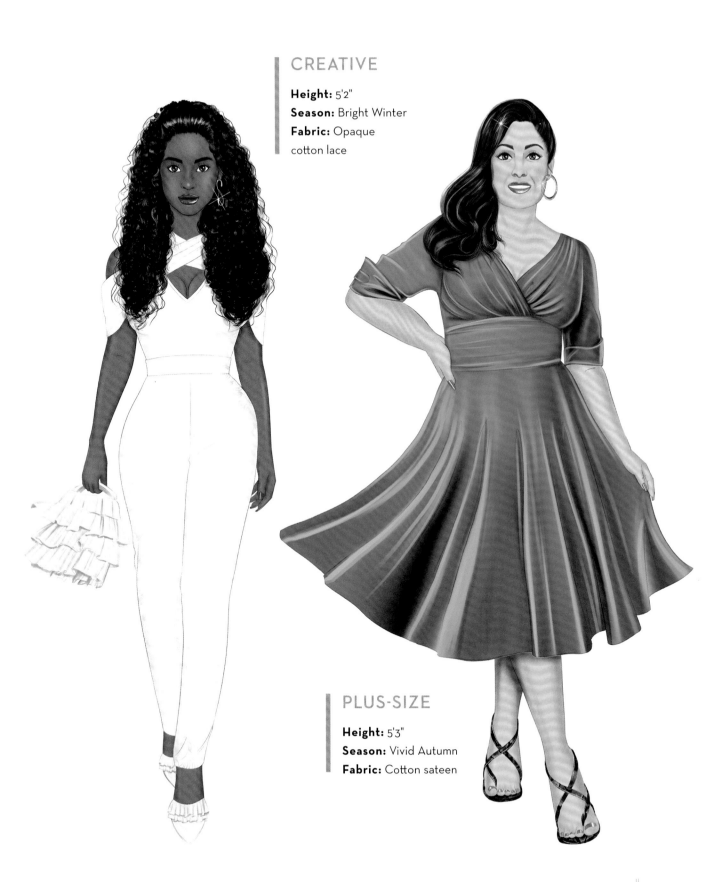

CREATIVE

Height: 5'2"
Season: Bright Winter
Fabric: Opaque
cotton lace

PLUS-SIZE

Height: 5'3"
Season: Vivid Autumn
Fabric: Cotton sateen

THEATRICAL ROMANTIC

LA FEMME FATALE

YIN/YANG BALANCE: YIN, with a yang undercurrent

LINE: CURVE + NARROW (height: under five foot six)

SILHOUETTE: You need a shapely outline that allows for and accommodates your curves. When one is looking at you, the eye needs to travel around them. It can be more fitted or more fluid, but the curves need to always be evident.

ICON: Vivien Leigh

EXEMPLARS: Dorothy Dandridge, Dolores del Río, Sharmila Tagore, Maylia Fong

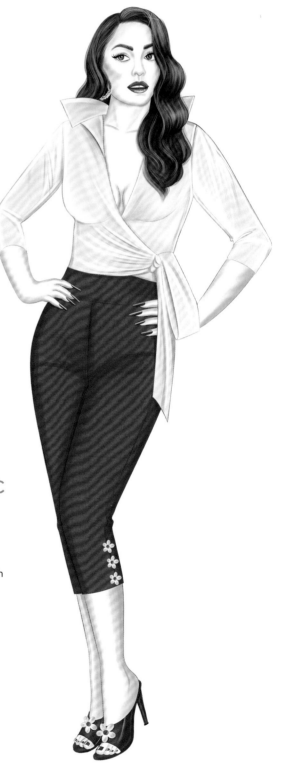

UPDATED ICONIC

Height: 5'2"
Season: Fiery Autumn
Fabric: Blouse: Silk charmeuse; toreadors: stretch cotton blend

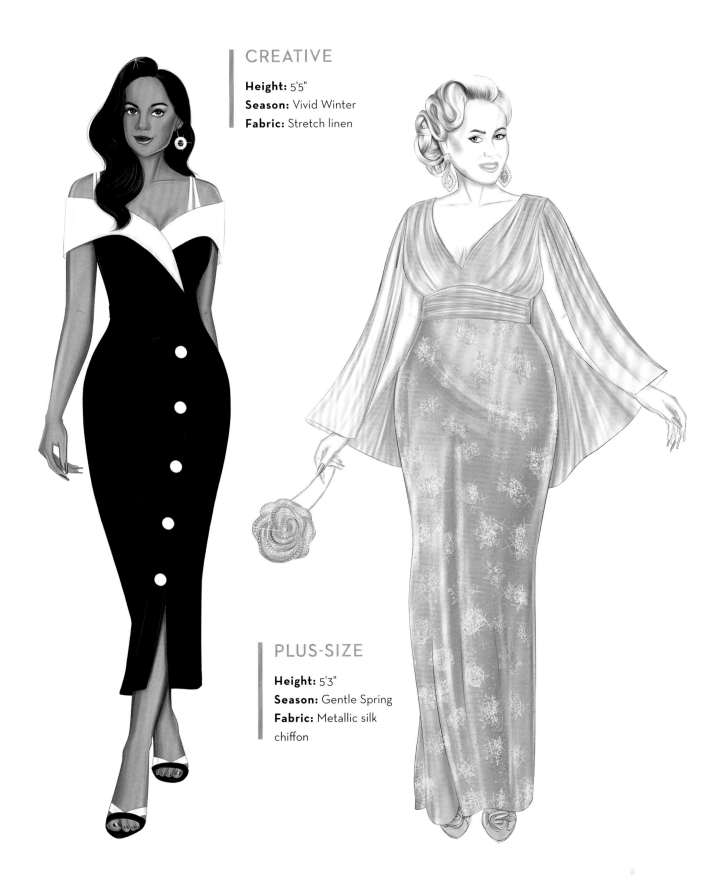

CREATIVE

Height: 5'5"
Season: Vivid Winter
Fabric: Stretch linen

PLUS-SIZE

Height: 5'3"
Season: Gentle Spring
Fabric: Metallic silk chiffon

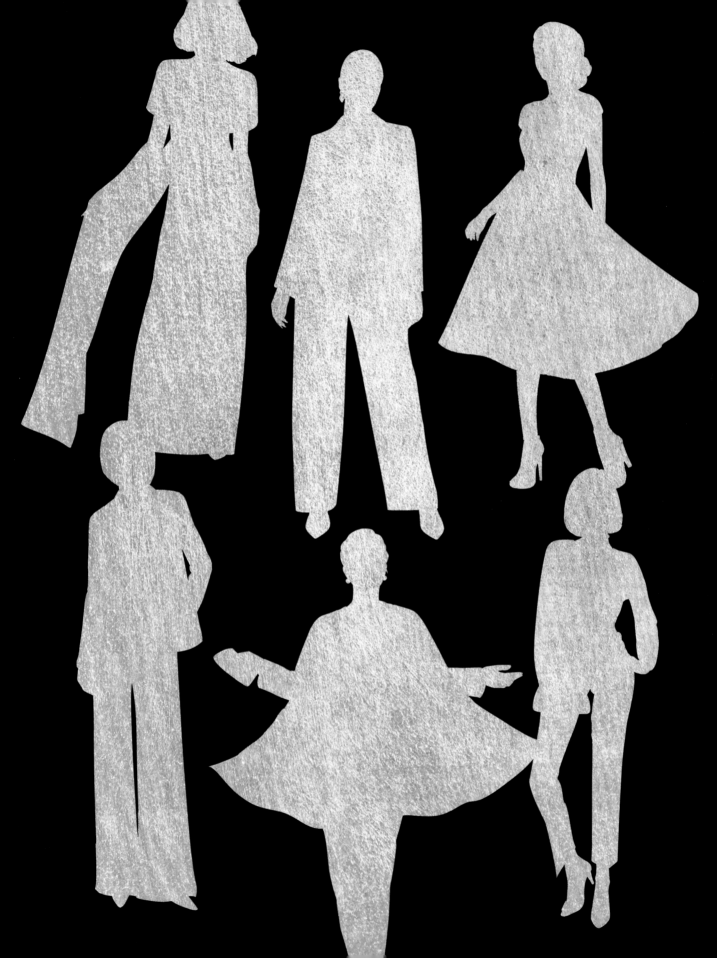

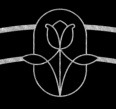

THE
CLASSICS

DRAMATIC CLASSIC

HAUTE POWERHOUSE

YIN/YANG BALANCE: BALANCED, with a yang influence

LINE: VERTICAL + BALANCE (height will be under five foot six)

SILHOUETTE: You need a clean, smooth outline with tailored or sharp edges. Nothing too extreme or severe. When one is looking at you, the eye needs to travel downward, relatively straight. Likewise, any drape or flow needs to move downward, not out. Keep it fairly close to the body, without being tight. Time-honored simplicity, with a fashion-forward skew.

ICON: Lana Turner

EXEMPLARS: Ida Lupino, Nancy Wilson, Michelle Yeoh

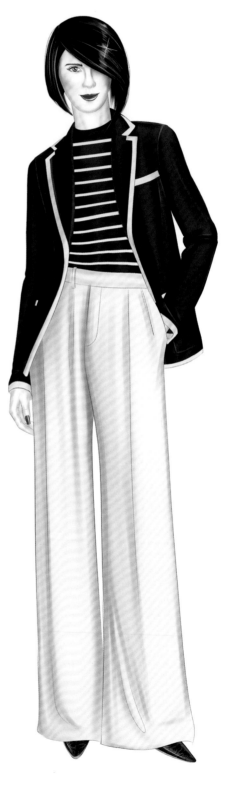

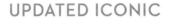

UPDATED ICONIC

Height: 5'3"
Season: Bright Winter
Fabric: Wool and cashmere

CREATIVE

Height: 5'5½"
Season: Vivid Summer
Fabric: Silk crepe

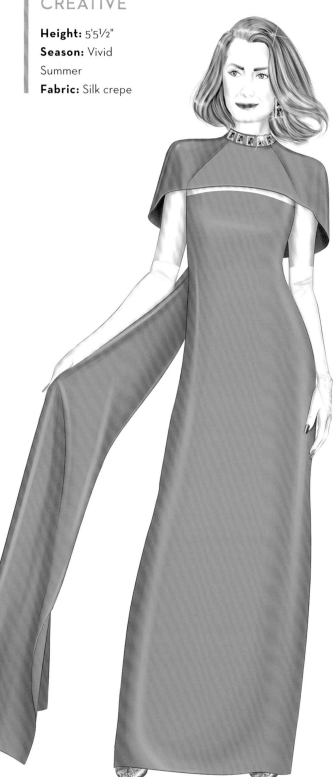

PLUS SIZE

Height: 5'4"
Season: Gentle Autumn
Fabric: Raw silk

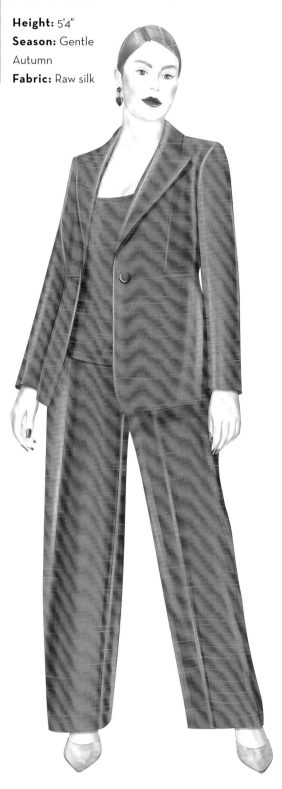

SOFT CLASSIC

HAUTE ELÉGANTE

YIN/YANG BALANCE: BALANCED, with a yin
influence

LINE: CURVE + BALANCE (height will be under
five foot six)

SILHOUETTE: You need a smooth, clean outline that
softly skims the body. When one is looking at
you the eye will travel in a fluid manner, subtly moving
around the curves. Shapely without being tight.
Time-honored simplicity, skewed toward the stylish.

ICON: Catherine Deneuve

EXEMPLARS: Nina Mae McKinney, Lupe Vélez,
Nancy Kwan, Merle Oberon, Anita Page

UPDATED ICONIC

Height: 5'4"
Season: Dusty Summer
Fabric: Polished cotton

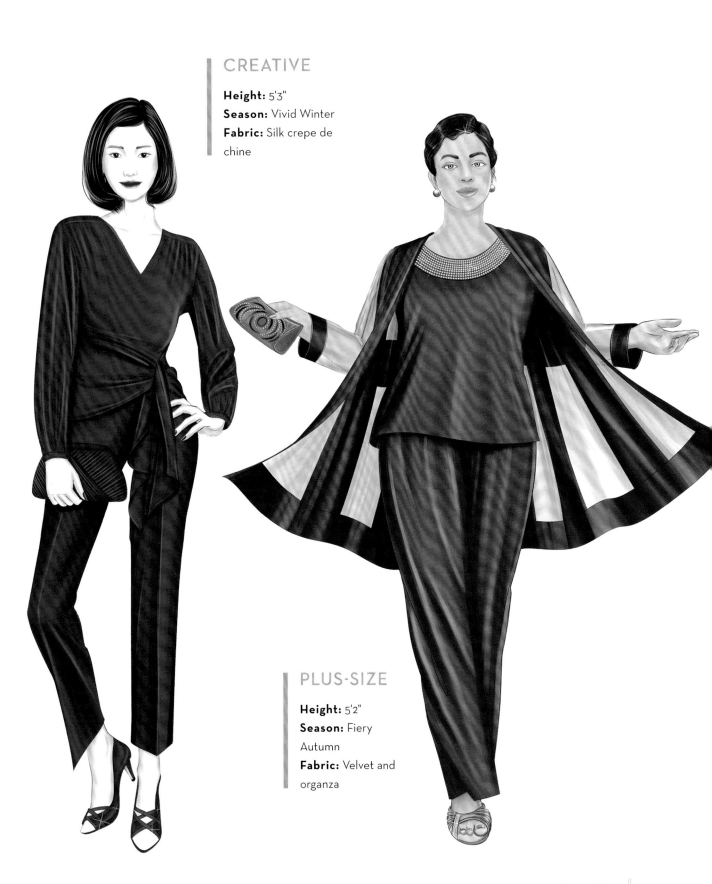

CREATIVE

Height: 5'3"
Season: Vivid Winter
Fabric: Silk crepe de chine

PLUS-SIZE

Height: 5'2"
Season: Fiery Autumn
Fabric: Velvet and organza

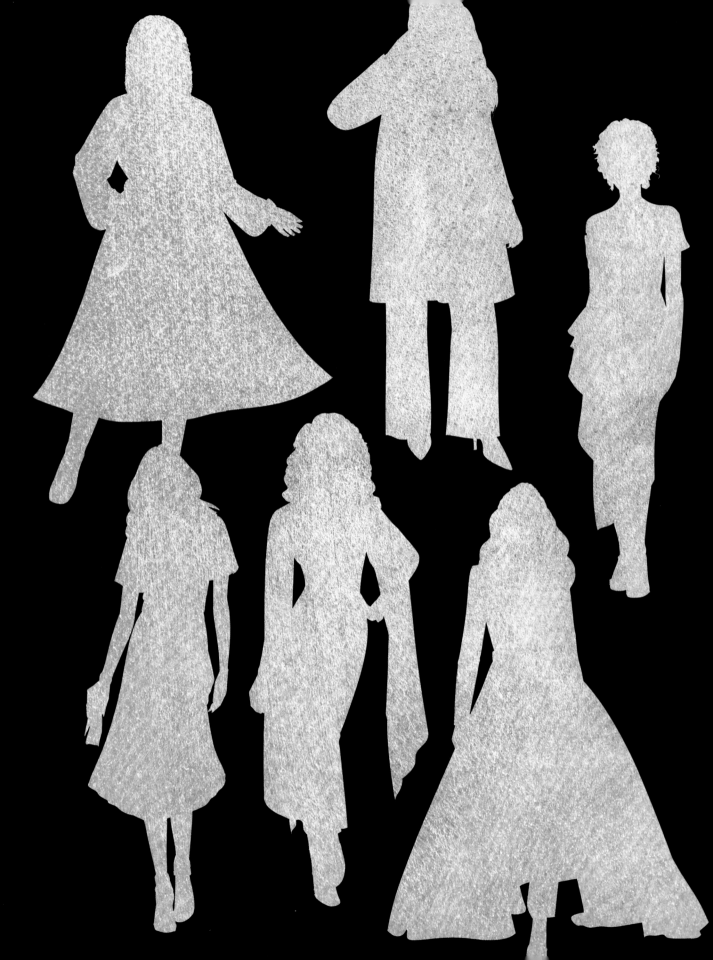

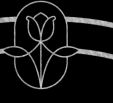

THE
NATURALS

FLAMBOYANT NATURAL

THE NONCHALANT SHOWSTOPPER

YIN/YANG BALANCE: YANG, bold, blunt

LINE: VERTICAL + WIDTH (any height is possible, but usually five foot six and over)

SILHOUETTE: You need a relaxed, straight outline that is long and unbroken, with breadth through the upper back/shoulder area. When one is looking at you, the eye will travel in one bold sweep moving downward. Any flow/drape should move downward, not out.

ICON: Mitzi Gaynor

EXEMPLARS: Dionne Warwick, Maria Montez, Josephine Baker, Madhubala, María Félix, Lisa Lu

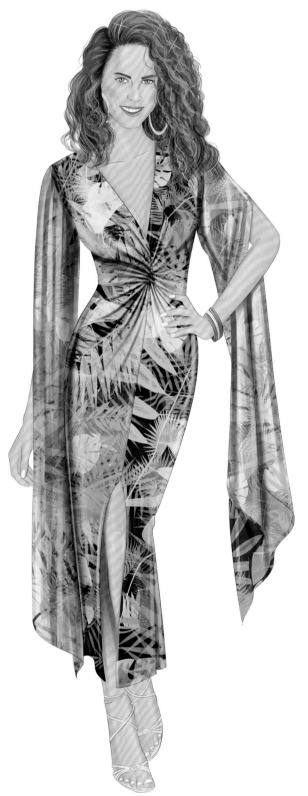

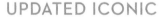

UPDATED ICONIC

Height: 5'7"
Season: Gentle Autumn
Fabric: Chiffon

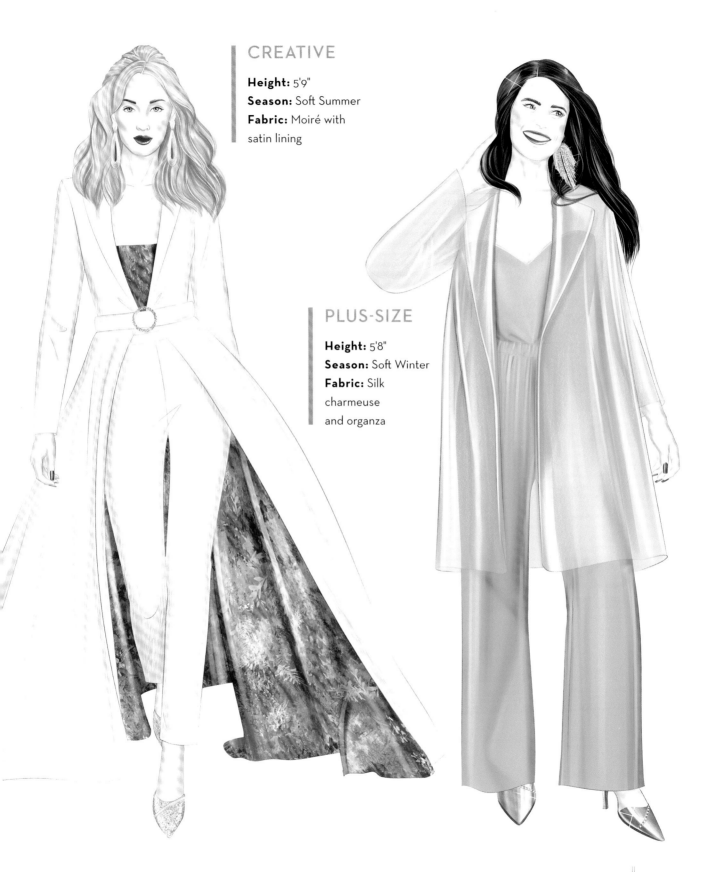

CREATIVE

Height: 5'9"
Season: Soft Summer
Fabric: Moiré with satin lining

PLUS-SIZE

Height: 5'8"
Season: Soft Winter
Fabric: Silk charmeuse and organza

SOFT NATURAL

THE SASSY COVER GIRL

YIN/YANG BALANCE: YANG, with a yin undercurrent

LINE: CURVE + WIDTH (height will be under five foot six)

SILHOUETTE: You need an outline that has breadth through the upper back and then moves around the curve. When one is looking at you, the eye will travel out and then around. Any flow or drape should reveal the curves but not be stiff or too tight. Nothing fussy for you!

ICON: Betty Grable

EXEMPLARS: Aretha Franklin, Dinah Washington, Nargis Dutt, Lupita Tovar

UPDATED ICONIC

Height: 5'3"
Season: Bright Spring
Fabric: Rayon

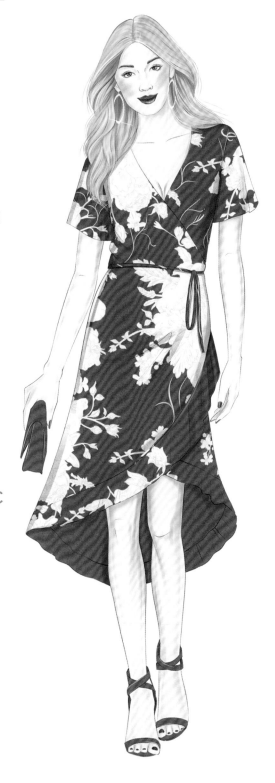

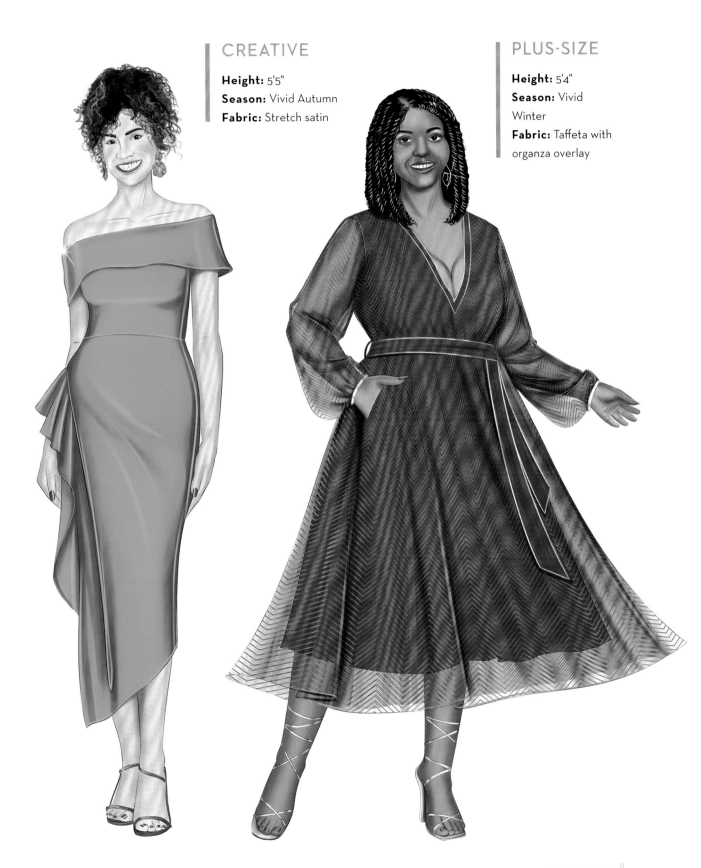

CREATIVE

Height: 5'5"
Season: Vivid Autumn
Fabric: Stretch satin

PLUS-SIZE

Height: 5'4"
Season: Vivid Winter
Fabric: Taffeta with organza overlay

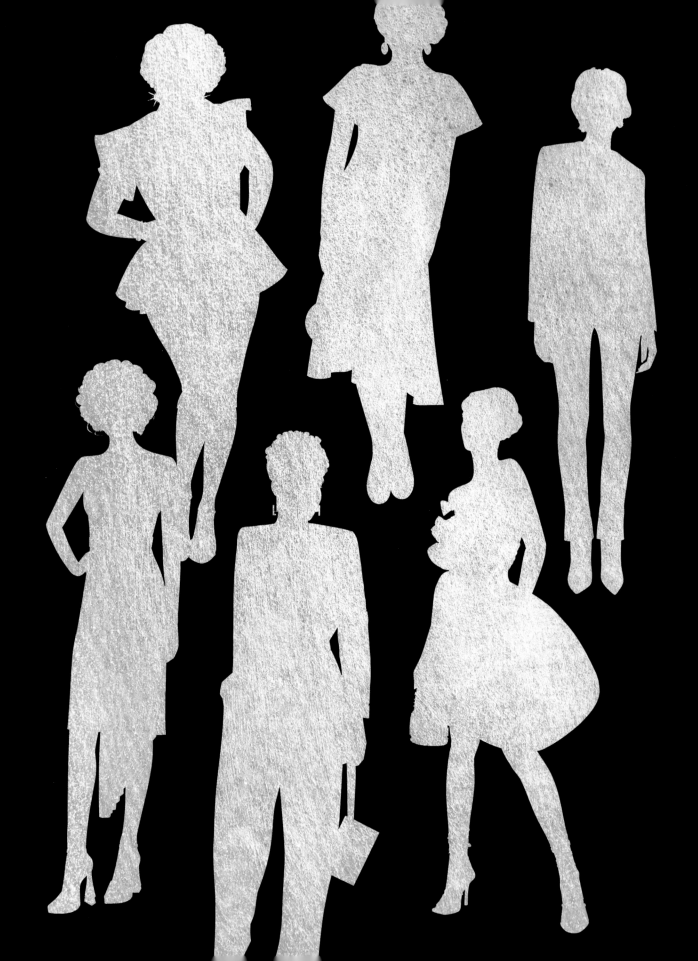

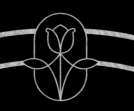

THE
GAMINES

FLAMBOYANT GAMINE

TRÈS CHIC ICONOCLAST

YIN/YANG BALANCE: COMBINATION OF OPPOSITES, extra yang

LINE: VERTICAL + PETITE (height will be under five foot five)

SILHOUETTE: You need an outline that includes a combination of two things: 1) a base of one long line moving straight downward close to the body, 2) on top of this, detail/separate pieces/accessories that add breaks to the base. When one is looking at you, the eye needs to travel downward in a staccato fashion. You need to keep your base close to the body. Any flow needs to move down, not out, and have the same breaks. Detail is crucial to your silhouette.

ICON: Audrey Hepburn

EXEMPLARS: Rita Moreno, Miyoshi Umeki, Diana Ross, Carmen Miranda

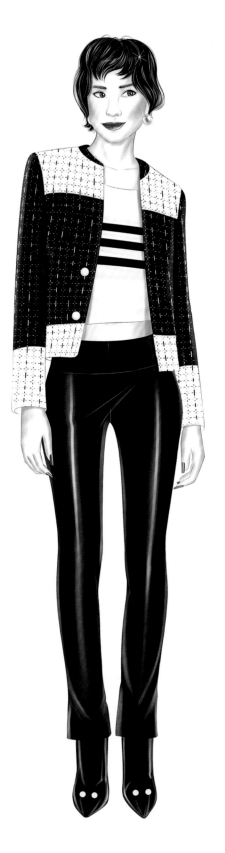

UPDATED ICONIC

Height: 5'5"
Season: Soft Winter
Fabric: Bouclé jacket, cotton T-shirt, leather pants

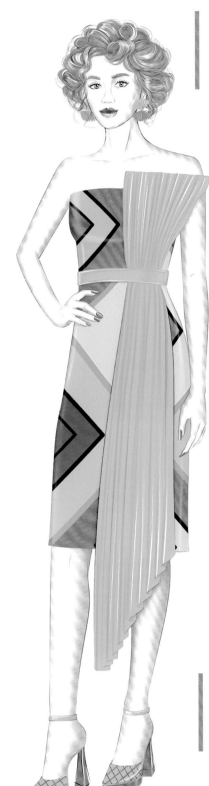

CREATIVE

Height: 5'4"
Season: Vibrant Spring
Fabric: Polished cotton

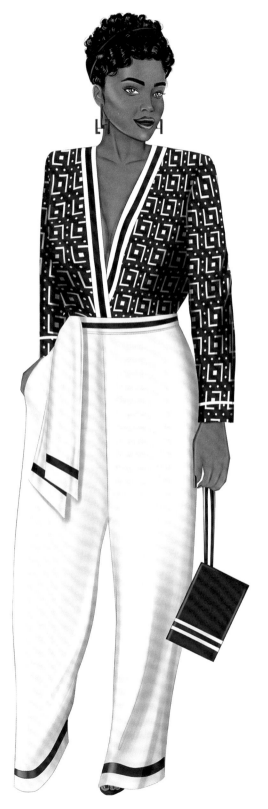

PLUS-SIZE

Height: 5'3"
Season: Bright Winter
Fabric: Rayon

SOFT GAMINE

TRÈS CHIC IRRESISTIBLE SPITFIRE

YIN/YANG BALANCE: COMBINATION OF OPPOSITES, extra yin

LINE: CURVE + PETITE (height will be under five foot five)

SILHOUETTE: You need an outline that includes a combination of two things: 1) a base of one line that moves around your curves, 2) on top of this you need detail/separate pieces that add breaks to that base. When one is looking at you, the eye needs to travel around your curves in a staccato fashion. Any flow needs to move outward, like a flounce, adding the same breaks. Detail is crucial to your silhouette.

ICON: Leslie Caron

EXEMPLARS: Eartha Kitt, Clara Bow, Lupe Vélez

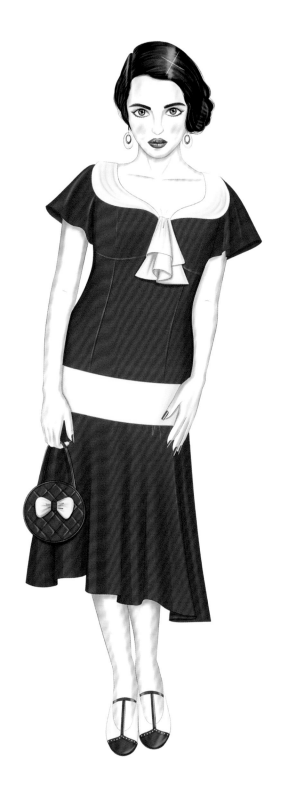

UPDATED ICONIC

Height: 5'
Season: Soft Winter
Fabric: Rayon

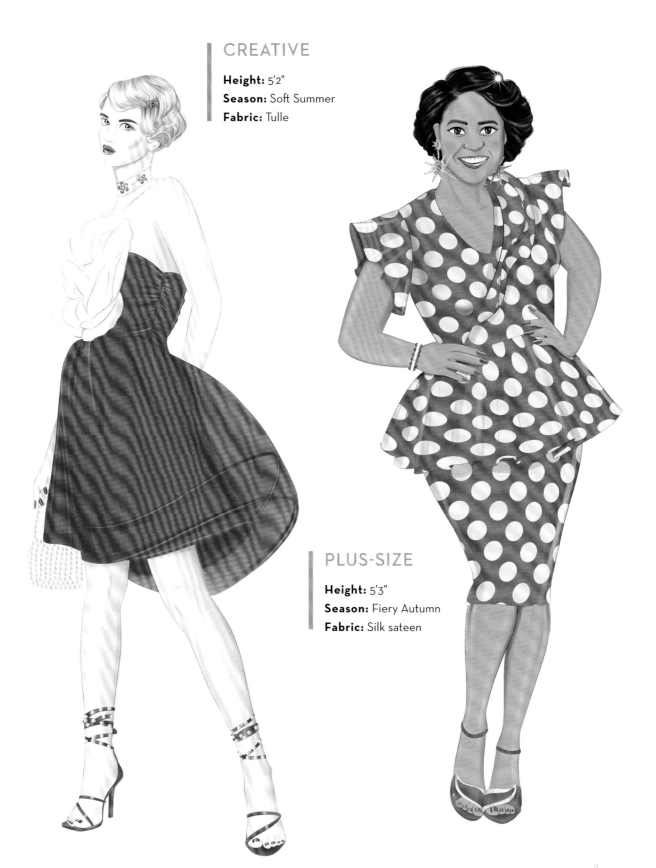

CREATIVE

Height: 5'2"
Season: Soft Summer
Fabric: Tulle

PLUS-SIZE

Height: 5'3"
Season: Fiery Autumn
Fabric: Silk sateen

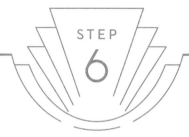

COLOR

YOUR TECHNICOLOR DREAMS

> *Color is a power which directly influences the soul.*
>
> —WASSILY KANDINSKY

> *Color is the language of dreams.*
>
> —PAUL GAUGUIN

I've had a love affair with color my entire life! Color is the magic of our existence. It soothes the soul and has the power to make us swoon. We *sigh* at the opalescence of a full moon. We *ignite* at the magnificent fire of a sunset. We *marvel* at the sparkle of a turquoise sea. We *delight* at the delirious riot of a field of tulips. It has always inspired, uplifted, and spun JOY. The way we process color is instinctive. We FEEL it. It is EMOTIONAL. It is VISCERAL.

Color, as well as all life, is, at its core, *energy*. We could further define this energy as the rhythm of life!

Everything in the universe *vibrates* to its own rhythm. The two primal rhythms of every human on this planet are: 1) our breath, and 2) our heartbeat. Our emotions all influence, increase, and constantly drive our rate of vibration, changing the rate of our breathing and our pulsating heart. We all vibrate uniquely, every second we are alive.

The awe-inspiring thing is, through our collective vibrations, we also interconnect with one another AND all the elements of the universe. This is, in fact, part of the whole basis of what Einstein called "quantum physics." *(Case in point: We've already marveled at our primal alliance with the stars!)*

Color along with music are the two direct links to our divine self. They both reach across all divisions of our world. They both speak a universal language based on beauty and love.

We don't need words to rhapsodize over a sublime Monet or to resonate with a thundering movement in a Beethoven symphony! *Just by experiencing,* they set our pulse beating and our breath quickening! They are both like instantaneous transports to the creative source of life itself.

Well, you have the same power to set hearts aflutter as any Rembrandt. It's called: THE MAGIC OF YOUR COLORING!

Since we've already discovered the power of

FORM by way of your sculpture, let's now unlock the MAGIC of your "painting" via COLOR.

Each of us is a *masterpiece of color*. Nature has given us a combination of complexion, hair, and eye that is not only equal to the greatest masterworks but also is actually the inspiration from which they were derived!

MONA LISA WAS A WOMAN!

Where do you think da Vinci got his inspiration for his masterpiece? What about John Singer Sargent's *Madame X*? Even the great religious artworks of the Madonnas are based on *actual human beings*! The rich and glorious colors in these pieces are simply evocations of what the models *actually possessed*!

You are the embodiment of one of the greatest crowning achievements created by the original and ultimate master artist: Mother Nature. If we can just harness the unique combination with which you've been blessed, we can continue the work nature began upon sending you to this planet.

EACH OF US IS A MASTERPIECE OF COLOR!

MY JOURNEY WITH COLOR

> *Try to be a rainbow in someone's cloud.*
> —MAYA ANGELOU

Let me begin with sharing my own personal color *epiphanies and evolutions*!

I've been a color evangelist ever since I can remember. From early elementary school all the way up through my current professional life, I have been both the grateful recipient as well as the ardent maven spreading the gospel of color to all who would listen!

I was first awakened to the fact that I had a special affinity and unique gift in this area back in third grade, when I was about eight years old.

At my elementary school, we had what was called a roving art teacher. We didn't have a regular art class until high school, but about once a month, we tykes were privileged to have the regional maestro come and give us a welcome respite from our usual readin', ritin', and 'rithmetic!

Luckily, our emancipator was a tremendous art docent! She had studied in Paris and lived and worked all over the world as both a painter and a teacher. Worldly, wise, and quite a character, she was both formidable as well as a whole lot of fun!

Visually, she was the perfect prototype of an art warhorse. Rather stout and possessing an unmistakable *basso voce,* she always sported this big plaid smock that completely covered her clothes. Hands in pockets, she would stride around the room, leaning over to proffer instructions as we would paint, draw, and sometimes sculpt.

The day that has stuck with me all these years, we were painting in what we were told was "the abstract form," which basically meant blobs of color! She came to me, picked up my "creation," and holding it up to the class, boomed out, "Mr. Kibbe"—she always spoke to us like little adults—"you have something special called an 'eye for color.'"

I didn't really know what this meant (except it sounded a little spooky) and probably would not have remembered this except this *color eye* moniker kept coming up through all my art classes and professional training. As an artist, I always had three areas that were considered where my special talents were concentrated: *color, design,* and *art history*.

In the early eighties, I was lucky to be in on the ground floor of Carole Jackson's Color Me Beautiful color revolution as it swept the globe. Carole was a wonderful mentor, and I quickly rose to the top tier, ultimately branching out to create the place I have occupied for over four decades.

To this day, I have traveled around the planet, preaching, teaching, and spreading *color love* to all who will listen! I have been blessed to be recognized as the go-to guy for color and have trained hair colorists and makeup artists from all over the world in my singular techniques.

Color is truly nature's greatest gift to us as humans. Nothing is more inspiring, enchanting, and delightful than *harnessing color in your life*. It brings joy to the world and truly uplifts the planet. It is your *personal magical power,* and best of all, through what we are about to explore, that power is available to everyone!

So let's learn how to become your own COLOR MAESTRO!

There are several properties of color that you first need to understand, before we get into the actual technique of what we will come to know as Seasonal Color Theory.

Just like with our Image Identity journey, there are basics you need to know about color before we can get to the personal technique of what you are going to do.

COLOR RELATIVITY

COLOR COMBINATIONS AND THE COLOR SURROUND

> *Colors must fit together like pieces in a puzzle.*
> —HANS HOFMANN

No color stands alone. This is the first thing I tell everyone as we start our color journey together. While we think of colors as singular, whether they be primary red, blue, yellow (or the various shades of these), color actually is never just one thing. We always are seeing color via what I call the color surround.

Let me explain what I mean. Suppose you are sitting in a café, and across the room you see a gorgeous lady sitting at a black bar clad head to toe in red, from hat to dress to shoes.

Now, you're thinking you're just seeing this lady in red, right?

Wrong! You're actually *taking in* a combination of colors: *this lady in red surrounded by all the colors of the black bar.*

If I were to move this lady and put her in front of a blue door, you would be seeing something entirely different: *the lady in red surrounded by the blue door.* Wherever I moved this scarlet lady, you would be seeing her IN CONTEXT of *red combined with whatever surrounded her.* This is what I call the COLOR SURROUND.

We always see colors in CONTEXT of what they are surrounded by.

Rather than "seeing" color, it would be more accurate to say we *perceive* it. Colors ALWAYS are taken in *in combinations.* That is why I say, "No color stands alone!" This is called the theory of COLOR RELATIVITY.

Color relativity is the first and most basic tenet of all color curricula that must always be included. Any color theory (and there are hundreds) must absolutely incorporate this as the one thing that is irrefutable. It is also the primary reason that Seasonal Color Theory exists.

Seasonal Color Theory is very specific and holds a singular and unique place in the plethora of color theories that abound. There are a multitude of color theories, each one valid within its own universe. Some overlap, some contradict, and some are relevant to specific purposes but are not applicable to others.

For instance, there are theories that exist as they relate to the colors for wall painting. Because they are based on how these colors are perceived when seen on white walls, they do not translate at all into defining makeup colors, which need to be considered as blended into skin tone. For that reason, the paint chips which are indispensable for your home renovation are completely unreliable for choosing a lipstick!

All of these different color philosophies are fascinating to study and can be of invaluable help in understanding the principles they were created for. At the same time, they are not constructed to work with the specifics of a person's coloring. This is important to understand before we delve into the techniques here.

Of all the color theories that have been promoted throughout time, Seasonal Color Theory is the one and only one that *defines* a person's coloring and *connects* it to the way color is utilized in her appearance (clothes, hair, and makeup). It's this combination of DEFINITION of coloring and CONNECTION to the elements of appearance that is the key difference.

The method is remarkably simple: Identify your coloring in a finite form, and then express it with a cohesive palette.

HARMONY + COHESIVENESS = FOCUS

The thing that we are always striving for in whatever aspect of your appearance we are enhancing is one thing: FOCUS. At the end of the day, it's how *clearly we focus* the elements of you in your appearance that counts. This determines how well people can relate to you, and in the end, how successfully you tell your story!

FOCUS is how we bring your STAR QUALITY TO LIFE!

We are going to learn how to connect things in a bit, when we put it all together. (Actually, 90 percent of this is built into this method.) For now, let's take a deeper dive into the harmony aspect of how color can change your life.

COLOR HARMONY

HARMONY, NOT HODGEPODGE!

> *Why do two colors, put one next to the other, sing?*
> —PABLO PICASSO

Let's go back to our analogy of you being a painting. Since we know *the colors of you* are the cornerstone of your canvas, how do we successfully *add* to the work of art *you already are?*

Because, as we have established, *you are not a blank slate*! You have a glorious fusion of hues in your skin, hair, and eyes! This *combination of you* needs to be *honored* with *complementary colors*!

In short, we simply want to add colors that go with what is already there.

We don't want to fight or cancel out the great work of art nature has already produced. COLOR HARMONY is the key.

Picture, for a moment, one of Monet's ethereal landscapes. Now visualize one of Mondrian's primary jolts of geometry. Can you imagine a mixture of those two? They don't harmonize at all, do they? Or what happens if we try to impose a russet and bronze Rembrandt into the mix?

We've just canceled out the specific genius of each of these masters and ended up with a big hot mess! Or, as we might say where I'm from, *a whole lot of nuttin'!*

The moral of this is:

COMPLEMENT for COHESIVENESS, CONTRADICT and get HODGEPODGE!

The next step is to learn how you define and use complementary colors in all the elements of your appearance that use color: *clothing (including accessories), hair color, and makeup*. These are your artist's tools that you use in enhancing your painting.

(Now, again, this part of the color technique has this connection automatically built in. Right now, we are still learning WHY this is crucial.)

So, to repeat, first, we look to CLARIFY your painting (i.e., what color mode of painting are you?). Next, we ENHANCE your painting with complementary colors. The result is: the FOCUS of your specific masterpiece.

So, how do we do this? This where my Color Magique technique comes in.

COLOR MAGIQUE

SEASONAL COLOR REFINED FOR THE TWENTY-FIRST CENTURY

> *God created people in Technicolor.*
> —BOB MARLEY

I've been a devoted exponent of Seasonal Color Theory for over four decades, and I absolutely swear by it! Its power to capture the core of a woman's beauty and allow her to shine has astounded time and time again!

When clients come to us, I always start with color. It never fails to inspire and excite. It has been the basis for the most astounding transformations I've been privileged to design over the years.

While I am a firm advocate of the original form of this program, I've also refurbished it as the years have gone by. What I am going to introduce you to here is my contemporary version of the seminal theory, as I have clarified and polished it for our modern era.

What I have done with my Color Magique is much like the evolution of my Image Identity work. Color analysis is an art, not a science. However, all art has at its basis what I call an "artistic logic." This could be described as the core principles, the "building blocks" from which every particular art form is created. These things are timeless. A higher purpose, a cohesive structure, and the technique to accomplish these things are all part of every art form.

Harmony is harmony, whatever the decade, century, or millennium!

At the same time, all art must relate to the changes that happen in the world or it becomes irrelevant. After all, as we all know, *change is also a timeless constant.* (How's that for a bit of irony: *the timelessness of change!*)

And then there is the further paradox that is just as true: *The more things change, the more they stay the same!* So, keeping the baby while throwing out the bathwater is always rather important! (Just ask the baby about that one!)

In my many years of color analyzing (i.e., "doing colors"), I have had the heaven-sent opportunity to constantly evolve with my clients. I have been able to see what was working as well as what was not and adapt. I've also been able to move forward with the times as our world has thankfully become more inclusive.

My goal with color, as with every element of my work, has been to provide clients with the ultimate freedom of self-expression. Giving women the technique to put their potential into actuality. Smashing the boxes that keep women either chained to stereotypes or enslaved to trends. Breaking preconceived cocoons and releasing butterflies!

I've also watched the Seasonal approach become mutated and combined with other color theories that, to me, have mixed results. While I'm not here to critique, I will just say that if you have come across any of what some term as expanded versions, what I am presenting will offer you a *bridge* to the core essentials. These are required ingredients that you want to make sure you have access to. There is a power to the original that can get watered down unless certain foundations are kept in place.

So, while my approach is rock solid in the four Seasons as they were created to be, there are nuances that I have added to bring it into the twenty-first century. This is what I consider to be the heart and soul of Seasonal Color Theory, which I have put into creating Color Magique to usher the complete magic of color right into your world!

Without further ado, let me introduce you to the ins and outs of my modernized and refined (while remaining faithful to the fundamentals) Color Magique.

Seasonal Color Theory in its original form is a brilliant yet very simple concept. It flawlessly does two things simultaneously:

1. Uses the four Seasons as templates to describe your natural coloring and generate a palette that is complementary to it.

2. Organizes your complementary palette in a way that has an automatic color cohesiveness built in (automatic color coordination).

Let's take a look at what the original theory is based on and why it is such an ingenious design.

THE SEEDS OF THE SEASONS

> *I think that to one in sympathy with nature, each season, in turn, seems the loveliest.*
> —MARK TWAIN

The roots of Seasonal Color as a recognized color theory harken back to the early twentieth century. In 1918, the makeup visionary Max Factor created his Color Harmony principle of makeup as he was creating realistic products for actors for the burgeoning art of cinema. This resulted in his discovery of the four skin tones and the crucial coordination of complexion/hair/eye color as being the two bedrocks that comprise a person's coloring.

Around 1928, Swiss artist Johannes Itten, one of the early proponents of the Bauhaus school, came up with his concept of four subjective palettes, which he then used the names of the seasons to describe.

Seasonal Color Theory combined the basics from these two geniuses and created a unique method of enhancing a person's natural coloring in their appearance.

Seasonal Color as it relates to you is based on two things: the undertone of the skin (also termed the base), and the triad of skin, hair, and eye (also termed the depth). Once you determine these two things, you find your Season, which gives you a complementary palette to use in choosing clothing, hair color, and makeup.

We will soon go into how to find your Season and what you do with it once you've found it! For now, let me go deeper into what the two components are all about. (Remember, at this point, you do not want to be thinking about what "you" are. We are still at the explaining stage!)

MOTHER NATURE'S SUPREME OEUVRE: YOUR COLORING

> *Colors are the smile of nature.*
> —LEIGH HUNT

THE BASE

Warm vs. Cool

The base of your coloring is genetic. You inherited this. It's in your DNA and it doesn't change over time.

First, everyone is either warm or cool. This can be determined by discovering the undertone of the skin, which is either golden (warm) or blue (cool). Everyone, from palest alabaster to every shade of olive to deepest ebony, is one or the other.

Now, the undertone itself is not visible. In other words, when you look at a person, you aren't going to find any gold or blue on the surface of the skin. What you do see, however, is *created* by the undertone. This is why we refer to it as your base.

In this respect, your skin color is created in the same manner as the color of a piece of fabric. Suppose you have two scarves in red; one is a fire engine shade, and the other is cranberry. The difference in these two reds is created by their base. The fire engine is warm, with a yellow base. The cranberry is cool, with a blue base. What you are seeing is the shade of red, not the base that created it.

Let's look at how this base works in terms of your skin color. For example, let's take a medium beige skin tone. It would be either a rosy beige (cool, blue based) or a yellow beige (warm, golden based). If we travel to a deeper end of the spectrum, it would be

either ebony (cool, blue based) or mahogany (warm, golden based).

Additionally, your base (warm/cool distinction) is carried through in your natural hair color and, in a much subtler form, your eye color. The three are linked genetically. They are all either warm or cool.

To elaborate: Hair has a natural warm or cool base as well, and it is always connected to the undertone. For our purposes, we can divide hair into either ash based (cool) or red/gold based (warm). There are cool and warm versions of every hair color that exists.

Take dark brown, for example. You would have either chestnut brown (warm) or charcoal brown (cool). At the lightest extreme, a yellow blonde is warm, while a platinum blonde is cool.

With eyes, it's more the impression. If you look closely, you will find there are many colors in the eye that will mislead. For now, just think of the effect as you stand back. A gray green, for example, would be cool. A jade green would be warm.

Now, remember, these are just examples to help you understand the theory. Every range of coloring of skin/hair/eyes is created with this warm/cool underpinning.

Let me also reiterate: skin, hair, and eye colors are a unit. All are warm, or all are cool. They go together. This is just simply part of your genetic coloring—another example of the genius of Mother Nature!

The first step in discovering your Season is to learn whether you are warm or cool. (And don't jump the gun here in trying to figure out what you are; we will get to that, I promise! Just not quite yet.)

So, for our purposes: A blue undertone to your skin equals Winter and Summer, while a warm golden undertone equals Autumn and Spring. This is step one in discovering the beauty of your Season!

THE TRIAD

Depth (Clarity or Dimension)

The second step in determining your Season is the relationship between the hair, skin, and eye. This is called your TRIAD. Either there will be distinct differences among the hair, skin, and eye colors, or there will be more complexity within each element. It's called either CLARITY or DIMENSION.

Each of the four Seasons has a different version of its triad.

The Winter woman has CLARITY to her elements, sometimes referred to as *high contrast* between the hair, skin, and eye.

The Summer woman has DIMENSION to her elements, sometimes referred to as *subtle diffusion* between the hair, skin, and eye.

The Autumn woman has DIMENSION to her elements, sometimes referred to as a *rich saturation* between the hair, skin, and eye.

The Spring woman has CLARITY to her elements, sometimes referred to as a *light/bright contrast* between the hair, skin, and eye.

Now, remember, at this point *this is not personal to you*. This is just to lay out the basics of the system. Right now, we are just outlining the *what and the why, not the how*!

So your Season describes the type of painting you are. Let's now go into the actual color palette that is going to work in harmony with your painting.

YOUR GRAND CANVAS

THE PALETTES

> *There are colors we can't see, but they're connected to the ones we can.*
>
> —WAYNE SHORTER

So now let's go into the foundation of each of the four palettes. The purpose of these groupings is twofold: 1) to give you a family of complementary colors, and 2) to give you a cohesive palette where all the colors work together for clothes, hair, and makeup.

The absolute genius of the original Seasonal Color Theory as a technique is the way these two parts are built in! Remember when we learned: *complementary + cohesiveness = focus*? Having a correct palette accomplishes this automatically! By simply using your palette, you will have achieved both!

So first, let me lay out the format for each of the four palettes.

The very important thing to remember right now is that each palette is NOT a collection of your best colors. That is not what Seasonal Color Theory entails.

What each one actually is: A REPRESENTATION of the *RANGE* of your possibilities!

Each of the four palettes is designed as a complete family for its Season and includes versions of every color on the visible spectrum. Each is organized around its versions of the three primary shades, red (fixed) and yellow and blue (mutables).

Within each family there are literally thousands of shades! They include *light, bright,* and *deep* versions of the colors you have at your fingertips.

So, before we delve into what your Season is, let's first take an overview of each of them.

WINTER: The Winter family is composed of clear, blue-based shades. The heart of this palette is JEWEL. The three ranges include the shimmering gemstones, the palest iced shades, and the dramatic deeps. The anchor of this palette is SCARLET (bright blue-red).

SUMMER: The Summer family is composed of diffused, blue-based shades. The heart of this palette is LUSH. The three ranges include the powdered pastels, the opulent brights, and the dusty deeps. The anchor of this palette is RASPBERRY RED (plush blue-red).

AUTUMN: The Autumn family is composed of saturated yellow-based shades. The heart of this palette is FIRE. The three ranges include the blazing tropical rain forest shades, the rich bronze/dark chocolate array, and the hazy hues of the desert. The anchor of this palette is TOMATO RED (hot red).

SPRING: The Spring family is composed of clear, yellow-based shades. The heart of this palette is: VIBRANT. The three ranges include the joyous Caribbean corals, the brilliant reds and florals, and the sunny peaches and honey browns. The anchor of this palette is POPPY RED (clear, warm red).

So, to recap: What we've learned so far are the basic elements of what Seasonal Color Theory consists of, including its purpose and the rudimentary definitions of the coloring and palette of each of the four families.

Now we move into the fun part, which I applaud you for so patiently waiting to get to: What is your Season! And this is where the rubber hits the road, because *we have to totally redefine how you perceive the very idea of a Season!*

YOUR VISION IS YOURS AND YOURS ALONE!

> *Everything that you can see in the world around you presents itself to your eyes only.*
>
> —JOHN RUSKIN

Did you know that no two people see color alike? It's true, because the way we actually process color is dependent on the physiological makeup of our eyes.

What we actually *perceive* as color is light reflecting off the object and then traveling through our eyes, where it hits the back at the retina after passing through the lens. The retina is composed of what are called rods and cones, of which there are millions! *No two people have the same number of these, and they are shaped differently for each of us!*

So, what we learn here is: First, we each have a different physical processing of color, and second, we each have a different interpretation of how we *perceive* color. (This is before we even get into those good ol' *prejudices and preconceptions* I've been haranguing you about!!)

With this in mind, can you see the folly involved in thinking there's any possibility of objectivity in the way color is seen? Remember all the things we found out back in the Potluck game? We face the exact same biases in our color perception! What we need to do is borrow the same technique we learned earlier:

Replace *faulty vision* with Authentic EXPERIENCE.

What we *can* do is discover our own individual visceral connection to color: the place where color thrills us, moves us, gives us goose bumps! This is how we EXPERIENCE color!

The first step toward this is to recognize that we each have a better way of harnessing the power of color than dismissing hues by judging them! If we relegate certain colors to a pile of automatic "rejects," we simply keep ourselves trapped in inaccurate "color prisons," sad places where our refusal to embrace new ways of experiencing ALL colors keeps us trapped. If

we were butterflies, this would be akin to clipping our own wings before we learned to fly!

What I want to first do, before anything else, is help you fall in love with your own coloring and ALL the colors! I want you to find your thrill in each of the palettes.

So often, I hear things like "I hate orange, so please don't tell me I'm an orange type!" Or "I'm a serious person, so I certainly will not even think about wearing pink!" Another good one is "Green makes me look, well—green!" I could go on forever about these preconceptions that only keep people in the same *color rut* they've succumbed to.

If you want the full power of color at your fingertips, the one thing you don't want to be is a COLOR NUDGE!

As a great teacher I know used to say:

Argue for your limitations and they are yours!

I love it so much when Susan and I pull out a sublime outfit in one of these colors a client "hates" and watch the client's heart just melt! It is supremely satisfying to introduce a whole new way of LOVING COLOR in all its glorious array!

So, it's now time to LEARN TO SEE WITH FRESH EYES!

I am going to ask you (beg you if needed!), for now, to put aside all your color likes and dislikes! (I realize that is a heavy lift, but humor me here, please.)

After we finish, if you really want to go back to "I hate puce!," I promise I won't hold it against you!

Right now, I want you to forget anything you may have previously been told about color analysis, the Seasons, etc., except the definitions I've charted out above.

I want you to approach each Season with FRESH EYES and an OPEN HEART. This will expand the way you understand color in same way we opened up your style when we played Don't Fence Me In!

Each of the Seasons is a poetic mode of giving an ASPIRATIONAL view of each family. There is majesty and resplendence found in each of nature's seasons. This is the reason, after all, for the very conception of naming each grouping after a respective season:

Four Seasons = Four all-embracing palettes

Just as there is no limitation to the grandeur of each season of the year, there is only a vast splendor in each of the four families that I want to awaken your hearts to embrace.

To this end, let's create a little color mirage for fun and inspiration.

FROM THE HEART TO THE HEAVENS

Visualize the heart of each palette (*Winter—jewel; Summer—lush; Autumn—fire; Spring—vibrant*) exploding into a veritable fireworks display of its specific family.

Imagine it flooding the heavens in a spectacular array of its possibilities. The unlimited range of each seasonal family of color.

The following are images of the entire breadth each palette truly consists of: why we never want to put a lid on color!

THE 4 COLOR EXPLOSIONS

A NEW WAY OF LOVING COLOR IN ALL ITS GLORIOUS ARRAY!

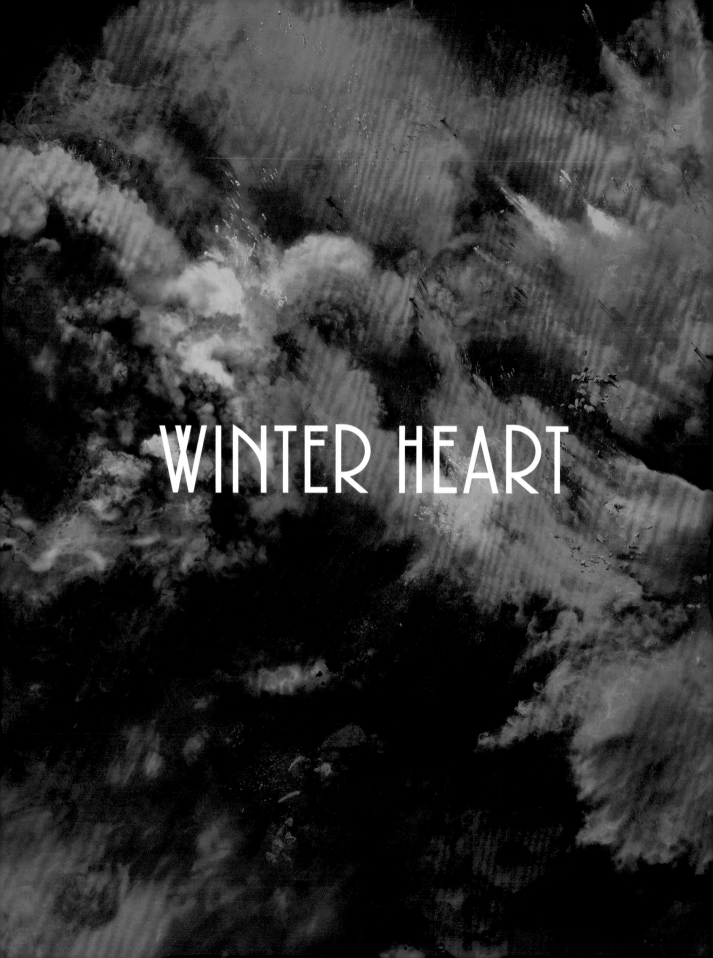

JEWEL

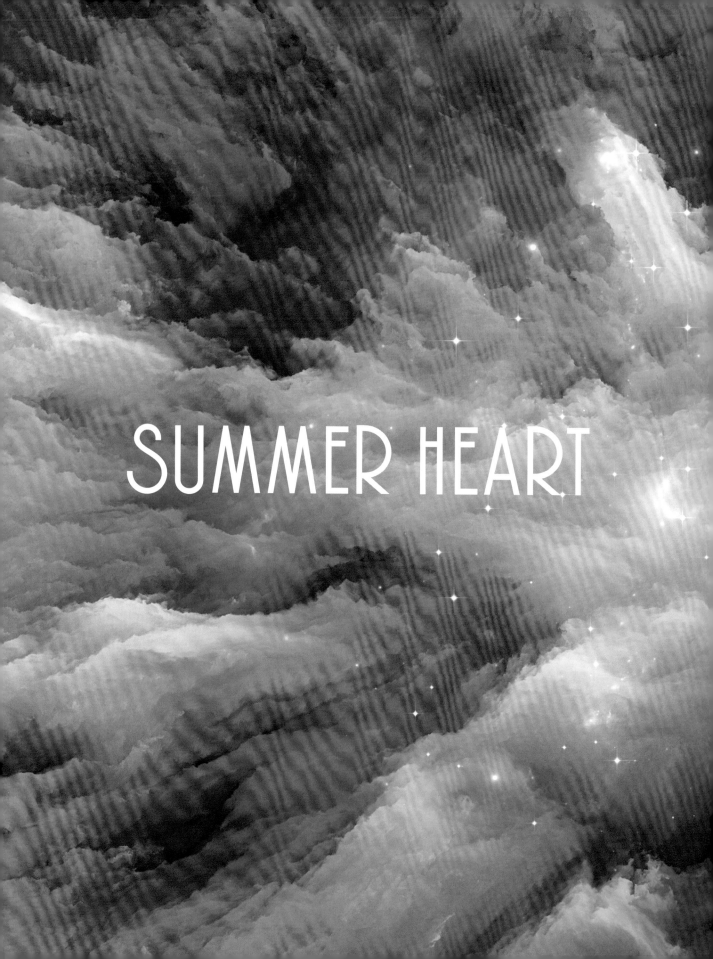

SUMMER HEART

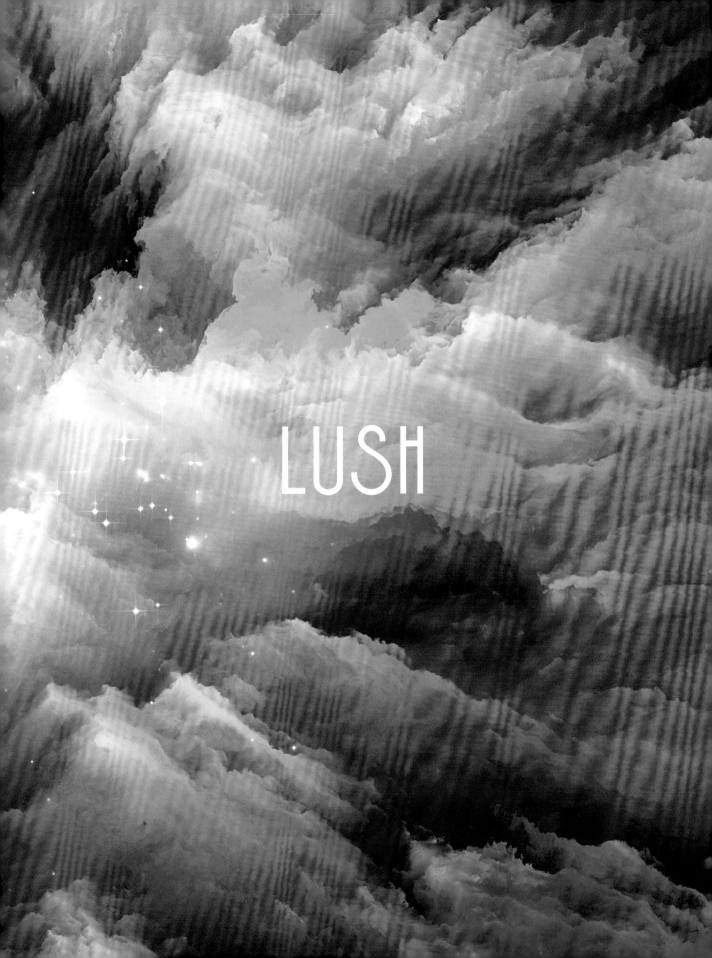

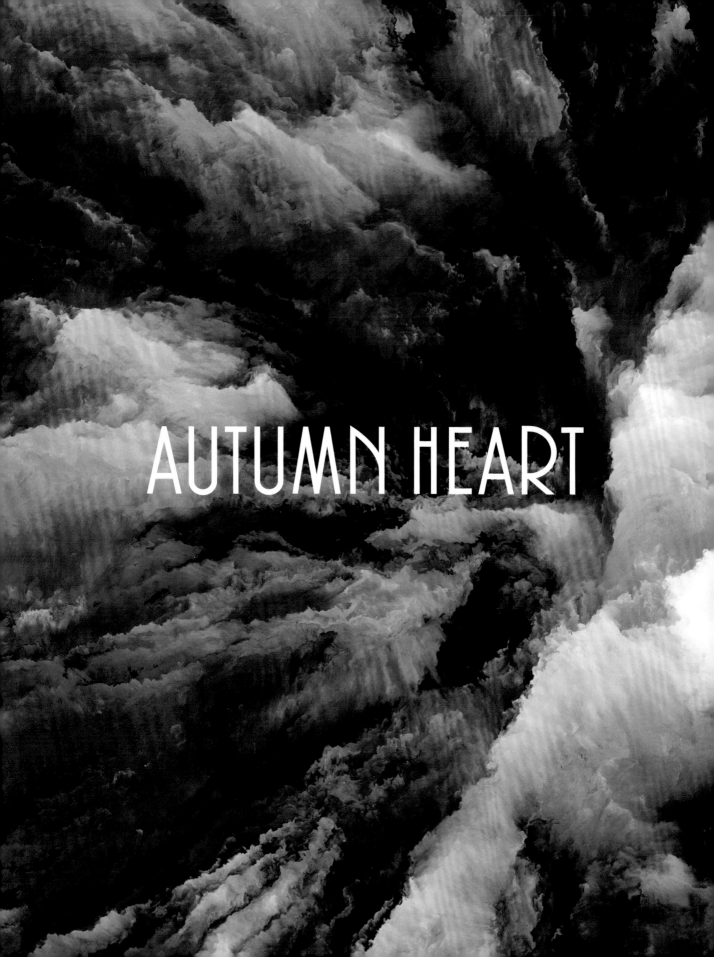

AUTUMN HEART

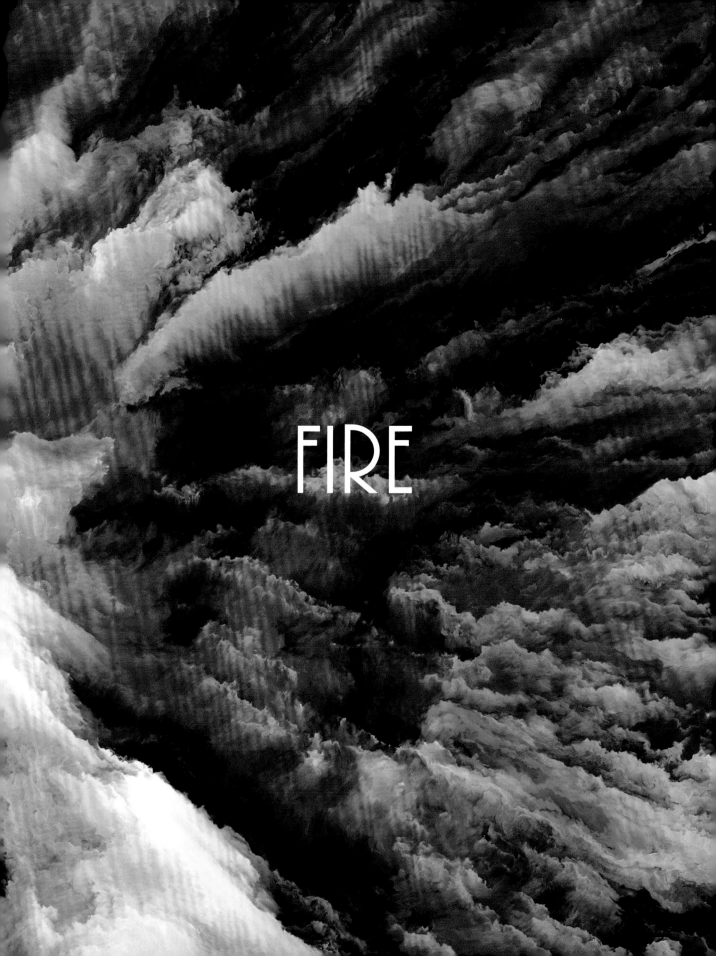

SPRING HEART

VIBRANT

BE STILL, MY HEART!

UNLOCKING THE SOUL OF EACH PALETTE

> **The soul is dyed the color of its thoughts.**
> —HERACLITUS

I want you to find one photo online that you feel encapsulates the heart and soul of each of the four Seasons. Put it in your online scrapbook site (Pinterest, etc.). Then below in the format, I want you to record a name for the photo you found along with its link, and also record the one word that you feel best describes it. (Don't repeat the "heart" term I've noted.)

There is only one requirement for this: Both the photo and the word must thrill you. Look for the ones that give you "gooseys," the "tingle," the "sigh."

Don't preconceive, just look for delight.

There is no right or wrong to this game. It is ONLY for you to find your own personal way of connecting to each of the four palettes.

NOTE: Don't forget to do your pregame warm-up (go to zero, pull up your awe, do Susan's Breath). While this only takes about thirty seconds, it will center you and propel you to the greatest results. Don't shortchange yourself by skipping your centering.

Here's an example:

SPRING HEART:
VIBRANT. YELLOW-BASED, CLEAR COLORS.

MY PHOTO: *A riotous field of tulips in Holland.*

URL: example.com

MY WORD: joy

WINTER HEART:
JEWEL. BLUE-BASED, CLEAR COLORS.
_____

MY PHOTO: _____

URL: _____

MY WORD: _____

SUMMER HEART:
LUSH. BLUE-BASED, DIFFUSED COLORS.
_____

MY PHOTO: _____

URL: _____

MY WORD: _____

AUTUMN HEART:
FIRE. YELLOW-BASED, SATURATED COLORS.
_____

MY PHOTO: _____

URL: _____

MY WORD: _____

SPRING HEART:
VIBRANT. YELLOW-BASED, CLEAR COLORS.
_____

MY PHOTO: _____

URL: _____

MY WORD: _____

Congratulations on doing something that has already changed your life! You have unlocked a key that is one of the most powerful parts of this system: **YOUR COLOR LOVE!**

I really want to stress how vital these two games we are playing in this section are to finding your Season accurately. There are so many preconceptions in the way the Seasons have been presented, as well as so much personal color prejudice that keeps people from even knowing what's possible.

The limitation of possibilities is, to me, the biggest crime that can be foisted upon the world!

So what we want to do now is *further eliminate starting with any of those color "I don't like's,"* and *replace them with a new vision of color surprises!* (After all, you don't really want to be a **COLOR NUDGE**, do you?)

YOUR COLORS ARE YOUR RAINBOW

When you approach the hunt for your Season from a love-based starting point, you have the unlimited spectrum of the entire rainbow at your disposal. While it's true that we only see seven colors in the heavenly arc itself, it actually consists of an endless array of shades! *It has been estimated that the human eye can in fact process ten million hues!*

With this in mind, let's take the heart of each palette to a whole new dimension and capture the entire unlimited rainbow of each Season.

YOUR COLOR PHANTASIAS

EXPANDING THE DREAM

> *You'll never find a rainbow if you're looking down.*
> —CHARLIE CHAPLIN

What we are going to do now is expand your "color love" into a rhapsody!

I want you to take the four hearts you discovered in Be Still, My Heart! and create **four dream boards,** one for each of your perceptions of each Season.

Each board should have between four and six pictures (no more, no less). Post these in your online scrapbook, and then give a brief description of the colors and any new, unexpected, and positive discoveries below. (Include your online link.)

Remember, there are no right or wrong images or descriptions here. These are just images that delight you that you relate to each of the four Seasons. (You are looking ONLY to expand your love connection here.) And don't forget to start with your three-step pregame warm-up to get centered. This will mean the difference between smooth sailing and nitpicking!

Remember first and foremost: This is a **GAME!** Have **FUN!!**

Here's an example:

MY SPRING PHANTASIA: _____

URL: _example.com_____

MY DISCOVERY: *I found my Springboard makes me want to jump with joy. My colors are bright and happy. Sheer delight. I've gone cuckoo for* **SPRING!**

RECORD YOUR PHANTASIAS HERE:

MY WINTER PHANTASIA:
_____

URL:_____

MY DISCOVERY:

_____

_____

_____

_____

MY AUTUMN PHANTASIA:
_____

URL:_____

MY DISCOVERY:

_____

_____

_____

_____

MY SUMMER PHANTASIA:
_____

URL:_____

MY DISCOVERY:

_____

_____

_____

_____

MY SPRING PHANTASIA:
_____

URL:_____

MY DISCOVERY:

_____

_____

_____

_____

FOUR RAINBOWS / FOUR FAMILIES

THE COLORS OF YOUR NEW WORLD

> *Life is a painting, and you are the artist. You have on your palette all the colors in the spectrum—the same ones available to Michelangelo and da Vinci.*
>
> —PAUL J. MEYER

We just learned that while a rainbow has only seven visible colors, there is actually an unlimited number of colors contained within it. Well, this is exactly the way each of the four Seasonal palettes is created.

Each of the four palettes is created as a *representation of a family of colors* that is connected via base (*warm or cool*) and depth (*clarity or dimension*). While each has a limited number of actual colors shown in the palette, it is just a guide to the full range of shades available to you!

One of the greatest things about color analysis is the freedom it gives you to create. Sometimes people fall into a rut with their colors and use them to be forced into a limited palette. That is something I hope to wean you away from.

We will get to how you use your palette to shop with and create fabulous outfits in just a bit. For now, just think of each palette as your *personal rainbow,* the family of shades that is your ticket to *color harmony* and your fast track to your ultimate goal: FOCUS.

The real potential of understanding your Season is the possibility for UNLIMITED CREATION. Your Season is your chance to explore the full range of your rainbow. You are not "light" or "dark" or any other preconceived label. This is why the rainbow is the perfect metaphor for creating your personal painting—ALL THE COLORS OF YOU!

The rainbow itself is a mystical symbol denoting perfection and completeness. In the Bible, it is presented as a covenant between God and earth, our connection to the divine. It is also a sign of beauty after a storm, of the hope that springs eternal in our hearts.

The seven visible colors of the rainbow are separate but run together. They are, in order, RED, ORANGE, YELLOW, GREEN, BLUE, INDIGO, and VIOLET. (Also known by the abbreviation ROYGBIV.)

Because the rainbow brings all the colors together, it also represents inclusivity and overcoming our attachments to differences!

Can you see how important this rainbow device is in our journey here? (Once again, that old "overcoming prejudices and preconceptions" rears its gnarly head!) You can't hate any one color, because each is inextricably intertwined with all the others!

Most of all, rainbows represent new beginnings and transformations. The rainbow that shoots high in the heavens is never-ending, just like our style is an ongoing adventure for all our lives! The colors of your rainbow palette are the unlimited colors of your life! So, let's first start by defining the RAINBOW OF EACH SEASON, and then we will define each of the FOUR RAINBOW PALETTES.

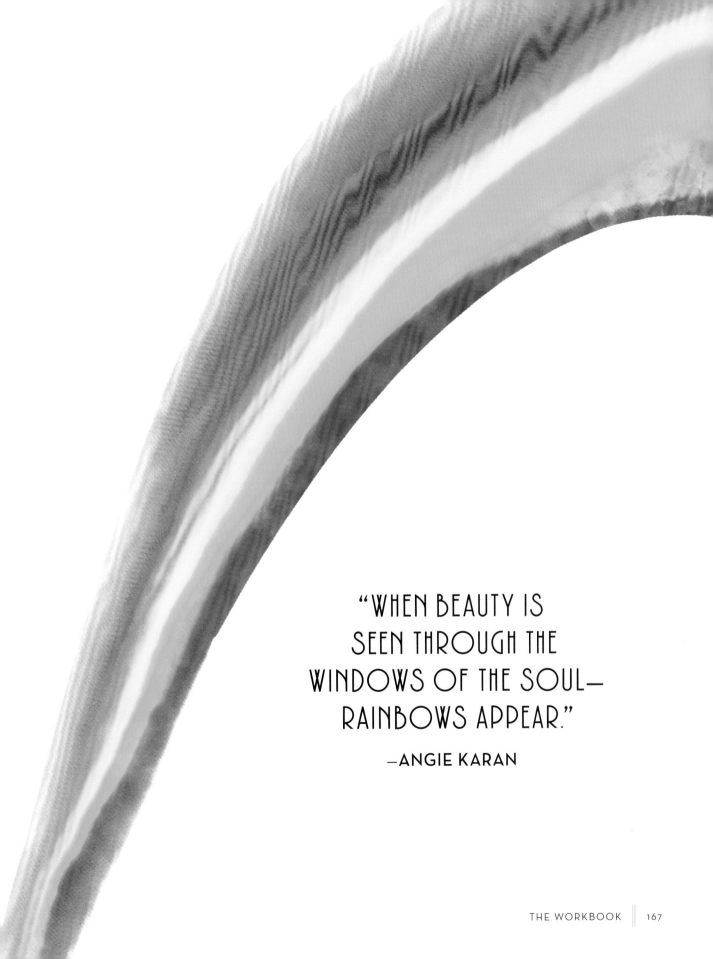

"WHEN BEAUTY IS
SEEN THROUGH THE
WINDOWS OF THE SOUL—
RAINBOWS APPEAR."

—ANGIE KARAN

THE *JEWEL RAINBOW* OF WINTER:
THE CLEAR, BLUE-BASED ARC

R: SCARLET

O: HOT PINK

Y: LEMON

G: EMERALD

B: SAPPHIRE

I: ROYAL PURPLE

V: FUCHSIA

THE *LUSH RAINBOW* OF SUMMER:
THE DIFFUSED, BLUE-BASED ARC

R: RASPBERRY

O: WATERMELON

Y: LEMON CHIFFON

G: MINT

B: CORNFLOWER

I: PLUM

V: AMETHYST

THE *FIRE RAINBOW* OF AUTUMN:
THE SATURATED, YELLOW-BASED ARC

R: TOMATO

O: BURNT ORANGE

Y: CANARY

G: SHAMROCK

B: TEAL

I: PEACOCK

V: PURPLE

THE *VIBRANT RAINBOW* OF SPRING:
THE CLEAR, YELLOW-BASED ARC

R: POPPY

O: CORAL

Y: DAFFODIL

G: GRASS

B: COBALT

I: INDIGO

V: VIOLET

Each rainbow is the inspiration and blueprint for each of the palettes. You will have a complete family of about thirty shades. They will be your versions of lights, brights, deeps, and neutrals. They are going to be your shopping guide and provide the color foundation for your wardrobe.

When you shop with your palette, remember it is a REPRESENTATIVE of your complete range of colors—your FAMILY. Use it as a guide to ALL your possible colors. Do not try to "match." The color of clothing should blend into the palette.

THE COLORS OF YOUR RAINBOW PALETTE ARE THE UNLIMITED COLORS OF YOUR LIFE!

THE FOUR RAINBOW PALETTES

WINTER RAINBOW PALETTE (JEWEL)

The Winter palette is composed of clear, blue-based (cool) shades ranging from pale ices, to brilliant brights, to sharp deeps. Your best metal tone is silver.

This family is vivid and festive, with drama and boldness making it a featured palette of Mondrian as well as the inspiration for the most famous jewels in history.

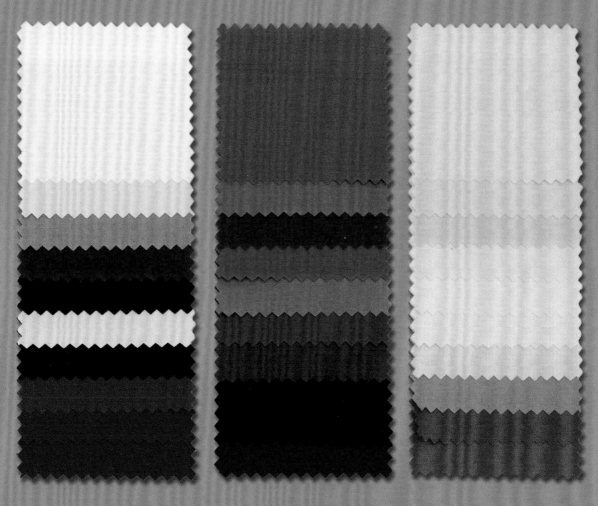

WHITES: Pure white, soft white

GRAYS: Clear, light, medium, and charcoal

REDS: True red, blue-red, scarlet, crimson, cranberry, cabernet

PINKS: Hot pink, magenta, fuchsia

GREENS: Kelly, emerald, spruce

BLACK-BLUES: Chinese blue, true blue, sapphire, royal blue, navy, royal purple

ICEDS (ULTRA PALE): Pink, orchid, lilac, lavender, blue, mint

NOTE: No brown. Avoid all warm or muted tones.

SUMMER RAINBOW PALETTE
(LUSH)

The Summer palette is composed of diffused, blue-based (cool) shades ranging from powdery pastels to dusted brights to smoky deeps. Your best metals are silver tones and rose gold tones. Do NOT think of your palette as muted; it is rich and sultry. It is the favorite palette of Monet and Seurat.

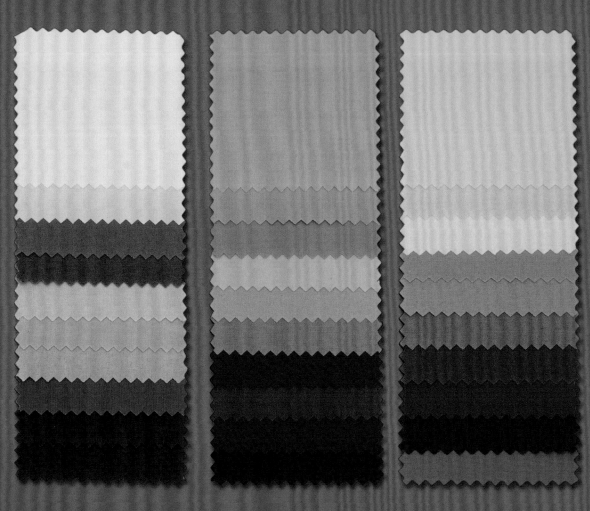

WHITE: Soft

BEIGES: Rose beige, gray beige, taupe

BROWNS: Cocoa, gray browns, rose browns

GRAYS: Blue-grays—light, medium, deep, charcoal

GREENS: Pastel, seafoam, mint, smoky spruce

REDS: Watermelon, raspberry, blue-red, cranberry, burgundy

PINKS: All blue-based pinks, from powder to orchid to bright

YELLOW: Pastel lemon

PURPLES: Lilac, lavender, fuchsia, heather, mauve, iris, smoky purple, plum

BLUES: Pastel, sky, cornflower, cadet, French, dusty true blue, smoky navy

NOTE: No black. No warm tones.

AUTUMN RAINBOW PALETTE (FIRE)

The Autumn palette is composed of saturated yellow-based (warm) shades. The palette is rich and vibrant, ranging from hazy to fiery to deep. Your best metals are gold, bronze, and copper tones. This is NOT a muted palette. The rich colors of the fall leaves, to the blazing tropical rain forest, to the sun-bleached desert are all contained in this family. Artists who used this palette brilliantly range from Rembrandt to van Gogh.

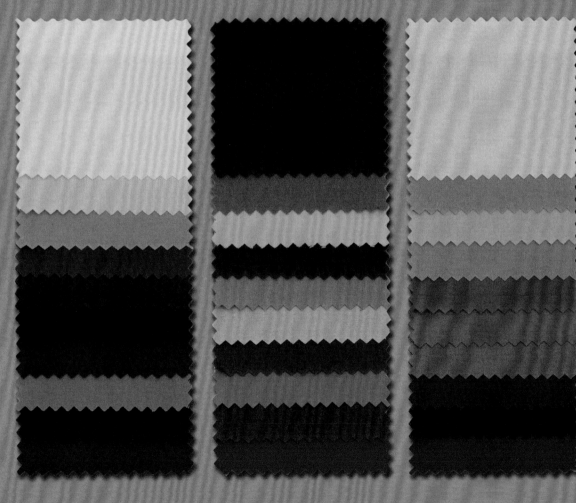

WHITE: Off-white

BEIGES: Warm, tan, camel

BROWNS: All browns, from golden to dark espresso, copper, mahogany, and bronze

PURPLES: True purple, plum, violet

GREENS: Kiwi, pistachio, sage, lime, grass, kelly, fern, olive, forest, pine

BLUES: Dark aqua, turquoise, teal, peacock, marine, navy

YELLOWS: Banana, mustard, marigold

ORANGES: Bright, burnt, terra cotta, russet, peach, salmon

REDS: True red, orange red, fire engine, tomato, brick, maroon

NOTE: No black, gray, or pink. No blue-based colors.

SPRING RAINBOW PALETTE
(VIBRANT)

The Spring palette is composed of clear yellow-based (warm) shades. The family is bright and colorful. It contains an array of light to bright to brilliant hot colors. Your best metals are the golden tones. While this family does have pale shades, it is NOT delicate. Springtime flora and fauna are the basis of this group. The more than two hundred flower paintings of Georgia O'Keeffe capture the magic of this palette of delight. I often refer to this family as The Smiles of Mother Nature.

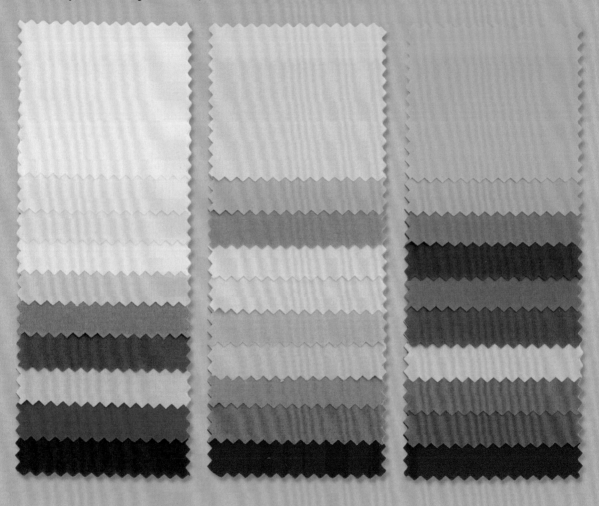

WHITES: All off-whites and ivories

YELLOWS: Sunshine, golden, bright, pastel

BEIGES: Golden beiges, from creamy to tan to camel

BROWNS: Golden, from light to medium

GREENS: Lime sherbet, pastel to brightest yellow-green, grass, hunter

ORANGES: Sherbet, apricot, peach, tangerine, cantaloupe, bright, warm coral

REDS: Clear, poppy, orange-red

PINKS: Hot pink, geranium, coral pink

BLUES: Aqua, turquoise, true, cobalt, bright navy

GRAYS: Light dove gray

PURPLES: Violet, iris, bright purple, bright periwinkle

NOTE: No black or muted or blue-based colors.

PRISON BREAK: ESCAPE FROM COLOR JAIL

> *Favorite color: I hate colors.*
>
> —IAN SHOALES

In order for you to find your Season, there is one essential element you need to define for yourself in order to keep you from making a major mistake. It's the most common trap people fall into, which, once discovered, and is really easy to avoid. All we have to do is identify it (with no judgment), and you can go right on your merry way to the freedom of your authentic palette. What I'm alluding to here are the colors you loathe, despise, or just don't feel you could ever relate to!

When I was growing up, a social centerpiece of the many churches in my small town was regular potluck. If you aren't familiar with these, they were dinners where everyone attending would bring their prized dish to this much-anticipated event.

Invariably, at the one my family attended, at the end of the last table—*the revered dessert buffet*—was: THE DREADED AMBROSIA.

This was the specialty of one of our stalwarts, a darling little lady of a certain age who had lived with her twin sister for what seemed to me and my friends for at least a couple of centuries. Convinced that her addition was so eagerly coveted, she would manage to send it over even when she was unable to attend herself!

Picture, if you will, a giant plexiglass bowl filled with a mixture of canned fruit cocktail (including the syrup), tiny marshmallows, and shredded coconut (the sweetened version), all mixed together with a viscous white substance she said was "that good whip cream from the box"!

She truly was a lovely human being, so no one had the heart to let her in on the fact that actually, this was . . . well, there is no other way to politely put it—revolting!

Just as I've longed to help you discover your love of colors, equally important for our journey is to discover the ones that give you a stomachache! We all have at least one that is our historical "hiccup" in our life: *our own dreaded ambrosia.*

These are roadblocks that can send us on wild-goose chases if we aren't on the lookout for them. My point here is to help you eliminate the biggest trap that keeps people misdirected in their search for their season: your "color yuck."

ELIMINATE YOUR "COLOR TRAPS."

THE YUCK!

YOUR AMBROSIA NIGHTMARE

This one is really easy, and you don't even need to do the pregame warm-up here because you don't need to get centered to do this cakewalk!

I want you to write down the one color that you just can't deal with! If mentioning the name makes your stomach turn, makes you flinch, or just gives you the heebie-jeebies, then that's our prize for this jubilee!

Pick only one color here. (Even if you find you have a couple, we only want the one that *irks you the most*.)

We aren't even going to go into the why or what for this. We will, however, be coming back to this as we get to the part where we find your Season, so don't dismiss this as less important. It is **VITAL**.

NOTE: There is no judgment in this. It is simply to bring this to the surface, so it doesn't stand in your way later.

MY "YUCK" COLOR IS:

SLEUTHING FOR YOUR SEASON

NANCY DREW, WHERE ARE YOU?

> *Women do better detective work than the FBI.*
> —KAY SMITH

To DIY your Season, you need to become a COLOR DETECTIVE! There is no quick-fix, one-size-fits-all method to find your Season except to have a professional analysis by a properly trained consultant.

However, just as in our quest to find your Image Identity, it is equally possible to find your Season, IF you remember it is a JOURNEY.

It will require you to, once again, *embrace your subjectivity* as a truthful and positive aspect. I want to remind you that your subjectivity is your greatest strength! And DIY is all about turning this into *intelligent subjectivity* until we reach the aha! of *enlightened subjectivity*.

After all, we've already learned about the way no two people see color alike, so how on earth is it possible to find an objective answer to your Season? The only way to approach this part of your journey is to realize it will take uncovering different CLUES to your coloring, one at a time. We will build a picture, bit by bit, that will lead you to your Season. But you have to realize that it is always going to be your subjective EXPERIENCE that does this.

So, I'm going to lay out several different parts to your puzzle that you will uncover one at a time. Don't be in a hurry to "get to the result." Rather, enjoy scooping out each piece as a wonderful new discovery about yourself! After all, your coloring is your painting! It was designed perfectly and magnificently by Mother Nature. She deserves to have you appreciate all the details she put into creating the masterpiece you are!

As we begin to unlock each of the pieces, it's important to remember that *this is not math or science,* it is an ART. And while it's not like learning a formula, all art is based on a type of artistic logic.

DON'T BE IN A HURRY TO "GET TO THE RESULT"!

DANGER, DANGER, REVERSE AT YOUR OWN PERIL

> *You first must be who you really are, then do what you need to do, in order to have what you really want.*
>
> —MARGARET YOUNG

Now, the first thing I want to do is save you from going down the rabbit holes that keep most people spinning their wheels and making big mistakes: THE REVERSE-ENGINEERING SINKHOLE!

The one way to guarantee incorrect conclusions is to start with COLOR ASSUMPTIONS.

These are things like *"I look like death warmed over in yellow"* or *"I know that fuchsia is my best color"*–type notions. Anything you are "sure" about, prepare to leave behind!

(Ah, here we go again with those dastardly p's and p's—prejudices and preconceptions.)

If you are going to be an effective detective, the one thing you must start with is a completely OPEN MIND. If you don't start with a commitment to looking at every possibility with FRESH EYES, you can easily miss the forest for the trees. (I mean, after all, Miss Marple never started by saying she knew whodunnit!)

THE DRAPES

So let's begin with a clean slate and start with what is often referred to as draping.

Draping is simply taking two versions of a color and placing them under the chin to see what happens to your face in each. Now, to do this at home, you can use pieces of clothing or any fabric items you might find at your disposal. (Towels, scarves, even pillowcases if you have fabulous linens!)

To do this effectively, you need to first assemble the swaths of fabric (or items) that you are going to use for comparison. Then you simply take one from each specific Season you are checking out and see what happens when you hold each one next to your face.

One will invariably make your face light up, and the other will make you blend into the fabric. You will want to do this in natural light, in front of a mirror, with no makeup on. Also, if your hair is colored, cover it with a white turban or scarf so it doesn't influence what you see. (I don't advise photograph-

ing yourself on your phone to do this, because the camera will distort your coloring and make any conclusions skewed.)

The only way this can be effective is if you follow a couple of requirements.

1. **KEEP THE SAME LEVEL OF INTENSITY IN BOTH COLORS.** (In other words, don't use one light color and one dark color. If one is bright, choose the other equally bright.)

2. **CHOOSE VERSIONS OF THE COLORS FOR BOTH WHICH YOU HAVE THE SAME LEVEL OF *COLOR LOVE*.** (Don't compare a "love" with a "yuck"!) Your goal is to select the best possible versions of the colors from both groups you are testing. (Go back to the Be Still, My Heart! game for these choices.)

3. **DON'T USE YOUR DREADED AMBROSIA AT ALL.** (Refer here to The Yuck! game on page 174.)

Avoid any versions of the colors that fall into your hate area! This is important!

Now, this will take a bit of time, and you may need to go back and repeat this process more than once. I also suggest that if you are someone who likes outside opinions, remember that they are only going to be coming from another person's own richly embedded *p's and p's* that they bring to the table. (In other words, take opinions from others with a big helping of rock salt!)

Also, remember that even at their best, the drapes are not definitive on their own! They are simply one CLUE.

Here's a chart with a list of what colors to use for comparing the Seasons.

WINTER	VS.	AUTUMN		SUMMER	VS.	SPRING
Cranberry		Tomato		Fuchsia		Geranium
Royal Blue		Peacock		Blue Raspberry		Poppy
Magenta		Persimmon		Cornflower		Bright Aqua
Black		Espresso		Mint		Yellow-Green

WINTER	VS.	SUMMER		AUTUMN	VS.	SPRING
Cranberry		Raspberry		Teal		Aqua
Emerald		Mint		Banana		Daffodil
Royal Blue		Cornflower		Russet		Tangerine
Black		Charcoal		Forest Green		Yellow-Green

WINTER	VS.	SPRING		AUTUMN	VS.	SUMMER
Royal Blue		Bright Aqua		Deep Peach		Mauve
Cranberry		Poppy		Purple		Plum
Emerald		Yellow-Green		Teal		Cornflower
Charcoal		Camel		Chocolate		Blue-Gray

Now, remember, even if you are positive you have blossomed in one of these groupings, this is just a CLUE.

THE BLUEPRINT FOR EACH SEASON

The following is a breakdown of the individual elements that are required for each of the Seasons.

SKIN: Pale porcelain, pale to medium beige, all olive tones (from light to deep), coffee, ebony

EYES: Dark brown-black, brown, brown-green, green, gray, blue

HAIR: Black, dark cool brown, medium-dark cool brown, silver, white

SKIN: Alabaster, light to medium warm beige, café au lait, russet, chestnut, mahogany

EYES: Green, brown, turquoise blue, hazel (amber)

HAIR: Dark honey (tawny), all warm browns (light to chestnut to espresso), all auburn shades, warm gray, warm white

SKIN: Porcelain; pale, light, or medium beige; almond; cocoa

EYES: Gray-blue, gray-green, blue-green, cocoa (rare)

HAIR: All cool blonds (pale to deep), light to medium cool brown, medium to light gray, soft white

SKIN: Ivory, light warm beige, honey, caramel, golden brown, medium golden brown

EYES: Blue, green, light golden brown (rare)

HAIR: Golden blond, honey blond, light to medium golden brown, strawberry blond, light warm red, dove gray, pearl white

YOUR SEASONAL SWEET SPOT

> *The magic happens when you find the sweet spot.*
> —SCOTT BELSKY

As you can see from the blueprints of the Seasons, there is a wide range of possibilities within each one. So, let's discuss *where exactly you will fall within the blueprint.*

The idea of identifying places within each Season came to me early on. As I started to evolve in my color work, I realized clients needed a bit of further clarification to help them integrate the full range of their palette.

For example, as you can see from the chart above, different Autumns might have coloring that includes honey blond hair, bright auburn hair, and darkest chestnut hair. How could they all exist within one palette of colors? Well, of course they do. But there is a difference in nuance that I wanted to make clearer. Not only for the clients' better understanding, but also for training the hair colorists working for me and for the makeup design I had begun to create. What would make things more specific, yet at the same time not LIMIT the full range of colors each client has the ability to rock?

So I began to identify the variations of coloring that exist within each Season. What I came up with was the three different classifications of a person's coloring that each Season comprises. These are what I call THE EXPLICITS OF YOUR SEASON. You will find yourself aligning with one of the places within the Season you have previously identified with.

Note: The hair colors outlined below refer only to your color as it fully matured but before "God's highlights" showed up. (Some people call these grays!)

DEFINE YOUR NUANCES— BUT DON'T LIMIT YOUR FULL RANGE!

YOUR EXPLICIT SEASON

WINTER

SOFT WINTER

HAIR: Medium-deep cool brown, deep cool brown

EYES: Blue, green, gray

SKIN: Pale porcelain

BRIGHT WINTER

HAIR: Dark cool brown, black

EYES: Brown, blue, brown-green, green, gray

SKIN: Pale to medium beige, light to medium olive, coffee

VIVID WINTER

HAIR: Black, dark cool brown

EYES: Black-brown, brown, brown-green

SKIN: Medium beige, medium to deep olive, café noir, ebony

SUMMER

SOFT SUMMER

HAIR: Pale to medium cool blond

EYES: Blue, gray-blue, gray-green

SKIN: Porcelain, light beige

DUSTY SUMMER

HAIR: Medium to deep cool blond, light to medium-deep cool brown

EYES: Gray-blue, gray-green, blue

SKIN: Light beige, medium beige, almond

VIVID SUMMER

HAIR: Light to deep cool brown, medium dark cool brown

HAIR: Blue-gray, blue-green, gray-green, cocoa (rare)

SKIN: Medium beige, cocoa

AUTUMN

GENTLE AUTUMN

HAIR: Dark honey (tawny), gentle auburn

EYES: Turquoise blue, jade, light brown

SKIN: Light warm beige

FIERY AUTUMN

HAIR: Dark honey, all warm browns (light to deep chestnut), medium to deep auburn

EYES: Turquoise blue, hazel (golden), green, brown-green, brown

SKIN: Alabaster, light to medium warm beige, café au lait, russet

VIVID AUTUMN

HAIR: Dark chestnut, dark auburn, espresso

EYES: Brown, brown-green

SKIN: Pale warm beige, medium warm beige, chestnut, mahogany

SPRING

GENTLE SPRING

HAIR: Golden blond, light strawberry blond

EYES: Blue, blue-green

SKIN: Ivory, light warm beige

BRIGHT SPRING

HAIR: Golden blond, honey blond, light to medium golden brown, strawberry blond, light clear red

EYES: Blue, green, blue-green

SKIN: Ivory, light warm beige, honey

VIBRANT SPRING

HAIR: Bright auburn, medium golden brown

EYES: Blue, green, golden brown (rare)

SKIN: Ivory, light to medium warm beige, medium golden brown

Now, a little sidebar here: Today there are many hybrids and mutations of what are labeled seasons, including what are called "expanded" versions with numerous "sub-seasons." They offer limited palettes that correspond to the names, some of which appear to be the same or similar to the ones I created several decades ago. While I am not critiquing these in any way, they are not the same, nor do they have the equivalent purpose of my EXPLICITS. My clarifications have the full range of the entire palette for each Season.

It's important to note that your Explicits are not assigning different palettes. To reiterate what I've said before, each of the four palettes is a FAMILY of color. Each of the four is a REPRESENTATIVE OF A RANGE that is vast. Everyone has the availability of the entire range to work with.

This is the genius of Seasonal Color as it was originally invented. It gives you the parameter of a complementary palette while allowing the full freedom of your individuality to flower! This is why it's so important not to be seduced into thinking about using it to dictate "your best colors." There is no such thing as "best" in color, because color is dependent on HOW IT IS USED.

Your Season gives you the blueprint; *it's your absolute prerogative to decide what you build with it.* Your colors are limited only by the unlimited frontier of your imagination and your heart's desire.

So, between the drapes and the breakdowns, you should find your Season. Some people's are more obvious than others', so don't despair if you need time to let this all sink in. It's okay to experiment for as long as you need to find your way through this. You will be amazed at how this can suddenly all fit together!

BELLS ARE RINGING AND TIME FOR SINGING!

YOU DID IT! YOU'VE FOUND YOUR IMAGE IDENTITY AND YOUR SEASON!! NOW LET'S CREATE THE MAGIC!

PUTTING IT TOGETHER

LET'S MAKE MUSIC!

> *Bit by bit, putting it together . . . Piece by piece, only way to make a work of art.*
>
> —STEPHEN SONDHEIM

Now that you've learned the major pieces, it's time to start assembling them into your "picture." This is how you actually begin to achieve your STYLE, which is both your personal trademark and your vessel of communication.

I want to remind you about our earlier discoveries of the NEW PARADIGM that outlined what your style actually is and what it does:

How you spread your message, tell your story, and share your light with the world.

STYLE IS YOUR PERSONAL ART, and like all art, it requires a comprehensible form in order to get out of your own head and blaze forth into the cosmos. It's not enough to simply discover your Season and your Image identity. We've got to consciously combine them into a form that is able to be made sense of by the world. That's where Love-Based Beauty comes in.

Remember in the beginning of our journey when I shared my early piano experience with you? I had the great fortune to have the head of the piano department explain that my fingers couldn't quite express my musical talent, and that I needed to obtain better technique in order to create what my soul had the desire to do. Once I switched to the master I was so fortunate enough to have been blessed with, I blossomed. It was the *putting it all together* that changed everything for me.

Style is the music of your soul brought to life! It needs to be expressed through the combination of notes, which form phrases, which, when put together, create symphonies! I want you to experience the bliss that "playing your music" fills your entire being with. So let's find out how we can give you the tools to make your "music" come to glorious life.

FOCUS, FOCUS, AND . . . FOCUS!

IT'S ALL ABOUT COHESIVENESS

In Style, your goal is: FOCUS.

Your technique is: COHESIVENESS.

You have to have *cohesiveness* to achieve *clarity*. You have to have clarity to achieve FOCUS. You have to have FOCUS to express your visual message. These are always going to be the foundations for your STYLE, the building blocks of *putting it together*.

Unfortunately, in today's world we have to work even harder to find FOCUS because social media has made everything so fragmented with its "pick and choose" way of approaching style. *The problem with pick and choose is that it keeps your visual message muddled.*

On the other hand, combining your Season along with your Image Identity is the beginning of the process that will provide you with the clarity that we are seeking. Now we will go farther to learn a vital step. This is the inevitable and ever-trustworthy technique that will transform your style and zoom you right to superstar status.

HEAD TO TOE (HTT)

> *And we were dressed from head to toe in love . . . the only label that never goes out of style.*
>
> —CARRIE BRADSHAW

What I want to introduce to you now is the concept of OUTFITS. Today, it's more common to just select separate pieces without thinking of how they integrate into the entire outfit.

Yet this approach belies the fact that people, without exception, see us in HEAD TO TOE form. You are a full-length human being, from the top of your head to the bottom of your toes! What you are NOT is a "walking head" or disembodied, fractured combination of parts!

So it's really only common sense that if you want to harness the true power your STYLE provides, you need to stop thinking piecemeal and replace this faulty premise with the entire-picture approach to your presentation. It's NEVER about the individual pieces of an outfit; it's ALWAYS about HOW THEY ARE PUT TOGETHER.

Now, I know there is a school of thought that thinks what is called HTT is a relic of the past, a 1950s approach to style that is "hopelessly outdated."

That's just flat-out wrong, foolish, and frankly disingenuous. Unless you are living in (or visiting!) a nudist colony, when you get dressed, you are ALWAYS creating an HTT.

No one goes out dressed in just a sweater, with nothing on the bottom! Or conversely, no one goes out in a pair of jeans (whether skinny, "mom style," or ripped) and naked on top! Likewise, you're going to be slipping your feet into something. You'll most likely be carrying a purse. Jewelry. Headgear. If it's visible in a long shot of you, it's part of an actual HTT you are always creating. You can't get away from that, so it's a complete waste of energy to pretend otherwise.

Now, HTT is not the same as "matchy-matchy" (which seems to get some people all wonky-donky)! It's thoughtful coordination that is the key. Not just slopping things together and calling them "on trend."

The real skinny here is that it's not a question of "To HTT or not to HTT?" *Instead, it's always simply whether your HTT makes sense or does not.* Cohesiveness is the difference between style and the misguided elevation of "hot mess"! It's either: clarity of YOU or chaos of hodgepodge.

Simply put, you can't get away from HTTs; they're an unavoidable reality. Therefore, we want to embrace them in order to reap the maximum energy they provide. *In truth, they are the secret weapon of your STYLE!* They are your starting points and your foolproof checkpoints along the way. If you start with the desire and intention of creating a fabulous HTT, you can bet the farm it will pay off beautifully.

The three keys to a successful HTT are: COLOR, SILHOUETTE, and SITUATION.

Now, don't get nervous on me here. I realize at first glance, this sounds like a whole lot of work you just don't have time for, right?

WRONG! This is exactly why I knew all those years ago, a new vision as well as a new approach was needed. Nobody has the time, or, frankly, the expertise, to spend it creating MGM-worthy ensembles for daily life. The kids, the spouse, the job, the LIFE . . . there's no Edith Head rifling through Joan Crawford's closet, waiting to deck you out for your date with Cary Grant at the Stork Club!

With all the options and deconstruction of modern life, it wasn't possible to sort through all the demoralizing "rules" and come up with any kind of personal style that elevated anyone's potential.

This is the reason for my creation of the techniques that resulted from finding the combination of your Season and Image Identity. *You already have automatic coordination of color and Personal Line just by following your discoveries.* All you need to do is to learn how to connect a couple of dots.

In truth, you are already doing most of these by default, but without the full power that will materialize from becoming conscious and deliberate. And I promise, these will become so easy, they will be second nature. Most of all, they will introduce complete JOY in the steps as you master them.

CREATING A COHESIVE PICTURE

When you walk into a room, there are two things people automatically take in at first glance: COLOR and OUTLINE. We do this unconsciously, in an instant. We also make on-the-spot assumptions from this first impression.

Harnessing color and outline to work for you are the first steps in creating successful HTTs. Your Season and your Image Identity take care of the complementary part. What you need to learn, however, is how to use them in creating actual outfits.

(A large part of this is accomplished via productive shopping, which we will soon learn the ways to nail your treasures! For now, let's assume you have the correct items to work with.)

To do this, you need to step outside yourself and look at each outfit you are creating on its own. In fact, when you are building an outfit, do NOT look at it on your body in a mirror or in a photo.

We'll start with COLOR. The technique I created for you is called . . .

COLOR PULL-THROUGH

(A.K.A. COLOR CHORDS)

COLOR PULL-THROUGH simply means taking one color and pulling it through in accessories and/or trim as a connecting factor. (It's possible to do this with two or even three colors as well, but let's keep it simple for now.)

Let's say you have a white cotton sheath, knee length, that has blue buttons. You could take the blue as your pull-through and do shoes, earrings, a bag, and maybe a shawl in this shade. By doing this *you've pulled the blue through the entire HTT.*

Now, if you had the same white sheath sans the blue buttons, you could choose any color you wished for accessories and accents, as long as you used that one color to pull through. (Let's say you chose red to pull through. You might add red shoes, a red clutch, a red bangle bracelet, and red and white earrings. You would have a white/red combo that could be fabulous as long as red was the sole addition.)

The result is that when THE EYE TRAVELS as you are looking at the HTT, there is a continuity. It is like having color purpose. This turns a simple, boring dress into a refreshing showstopper.

Continuity is also paramount for elegance, sophistication, and simply the unconscious message: *the wearer has mastered the art of her style.*

When you don't do this (choosing colors outside the innate ones), you have a jerky kind of traveling of the eye. This results in that muddled effect that is simply confusing. Visual chaos is not an effective tool for spreading the love!

(Now, we are assuming the dress and accessories are already perfect for you, as we would have chosen them with your joy, your purpose, your taste, and all the elements of your individual desires.)

Often, there will be multiple colors in a garment. It's the same technique. You need to choose the color or colors that are already there to use as your *pull-through.*

Suppose you have a wild print blouse containing lavish sweeps of green, orange, and yellow. You have already chosen the green for silk pants that go below the blouse. You might choose the green for the entire pull-through, which would create an elegant effect.

An alternate choice might be to pick up either the yellow or the orange, or even a combination of the two for a sassier effect. The point is: You always take something built-in and carry it through the entire ensemble.

It's also important that we go back to that point I made earlier about including everything that people see in a full-length shot. Hats, coats, and any accessory is a part of what is visible. So don't forget them or view them as inconsequential. Many a dazzling outfit has been utterly demolished by a ghastly pair of clodhoppers!

I do want to address the notion that is sometimes referred to as *color blocking.* On social media, this is usually used to describe the pairing of two or more colors that have no relation to each other. This is not what color blocking was created to do originally. The term was meant to include color as panes, which all had a connection via the outline of the panes.

Successful color combinations are COLOR CHORDS. They go together to create *visual music.* Just as in music, colors that don't go together create *visual noise.* Always remember HARMONY is key. Build your color combinations with that in mind.

It's especially important to remember that when putting separate pieces together, *it's the together that counts.* Otherwise, you are back to the *what's in your head isn't what people actually see* problem. You have to ALWAYS step outside yourself and consider *what the outfit is visually saying.* Do the pieces add up to a whole?

Which brings us to the next piece of your HTT puzzle, SILHOUETTE.

COMPLEMENTARY SILHOUETTE

IT'S A DANCE, NOT A PRIZEFIGHT!

> *Cooperation, collaboration, and coordination are more powerful than competition.*
>
> —HENDRITH VANLON SMITH, JR.

We've already learned your PERSONAL LINE is the key to knowing what is and what is not a COMPLE-MENTARY SILHOUETTE for you, and why it's paramount in learning how to create your Authentic Style.

Now, the key is making sure you know how to do this when building an HTT.

The most important thing to remember at this point is to connect all the pieces so they make one harmonious outline.

This is fairly simple when you are starting with a *one-piece base,* such as a dress or a jumpsuit. The silhouette is innate in the one piece, and all you have to do is learn to accessorize accordingly.

But what about when you are using separates? Today, most items besides dresses and jumpsuits are sold as individual pieces. Sometimes these pieces might be designed together, but more often than not, they are sold as *stand-alone* items.

This is a big bugaboo in our pick-and-choose society that social media does zilch in terms of helping you conquer.

Tops and bottoms need the same coordination as your color chords. Remember, the one thing you want to avoid is CONFUSION as your style message.

I'd like you to think of your tops and bottoms as a love match. (Or at the very least are really, really good friends!) And, as in any love relationship, there needs to be *clear and loving communication.* You are basically taking two or more separate items and seeking ways to connect them so they speak the same language.

United they stand, divided they brawl!

Too often today, tops and bottoms fight with each other. Who needs that? You want to spread goodwill with your STYLE, not incite more agitation.

When the two pieces are united in line and theme, they *trip the light fantastic.* When they each come from a separate universe, they are in visual competition with each other. (Sometimes this is more a knock-down, drag-out fistfight for attention instead of a smooth, elegant tango.)

Your tops and bottoms, as well as all accessories, should be like fabulous dancing partners. You can't have a blouse undulating in a sexy rhumba while the bottom is krumping a hip-hop, overlaid with a jacket do-si-do-ing a square dance! (Well, you can, I suppose, but unless you are six years old, we all hope you won't!)

In other words, don't aggravate an evening dress with a jean jacket and lumberjack boots and a slouchy pouch. Instead embrace it with something like a silk wrap, satin slippers, and a beaded bag.

Or if you are doing a tailored suit, don't insult it by forcing it to accept a sloppy oversized sweater, strappy sandals, and oversized hoops. Instead, consummate its longing for its companions and marry it with suede pumps, a leather clutch, and a pair of simple pearl earrings. (Ah, sartorial bliss!)

CONNECT THE PIECES—ALL OF THEM.

Today, there is a multitude of possibilities for every situation, but whatever your aesthetics, there is one constant need: *All the items in your HTT should speak the same language.*

To do this, you need a connection in theme, which comes from utilizing the third key in the building of a successful HTT:

CONSCIOUS SITUATION

> *Dream your dreams with open eyes and make them come true.*
>
> —T. E. LAWRENCE

Another thing today that has changed from the past is the rationale for the *"What do I wear when?"* department. In the past, there were fairly simple, albeit also pretty rigid, rules about what was "appropriate" for every situation. It might have been repressive, but it was easy to know what was considered "proper."

However, with today's more casual approach to everything, the art of using your style as a magnet is lost, *if you don't bring raising the bar into the equation.*

When you go out into the world in a haphazard way, without considering what impact you have, you have totally negated the power of your style potential!

If, on the other hand, you dress with a conscious decision to take advantage of, and upgrade, your specific situation, you will feel the change in energy instantaneously.

The thing is, you are ALWAYS *dressing for situation.* It's just that it happens mostly by default.

Let me ask you a question. Before you get dressed in the morning (or evening!), do you think about whether it's going to rain or not? Whether you need a coat, or a jacket, or nothing at all? Are you going for a walk in the park? A run? Are you having a meeting about a prospective business opportunity? A romantic evening?

If you answered yes to any of these, you are abso-lutely involving situation in what you choose to wear.

I realize that may seem obvious, but the component that is often missing is the question "What do I want to get out of this situation?" This is the secret power CONSCIOUS SITUATION has over dressing for a "default situation." *It's the magic that occurs when you bring* INTENTION *into your* HTTs.

CONCIOUS SITUATION means you deliberately think about the situation you are about to enter while at the same time asking yourself the question "What is my wish, from this situation?"

When you are conscious of your situation, you have the chance to add DESIRE and DREAMS to your style choice. This is how you begin to access the first part of the POWER of your style. (The second part being the inclusion of how it connects you to others.)

This brings us to our next three games. These are going to help you move away from today's lackadaisical approach to situation that keeps you in a style rut and keeps your life's aspirations on hold. These are going to help you EXPERIENCE the power that exists in you, which is dormant but just itching for you to harness!

They also are going to launch us into the next stop along our journey, which will ultimately make the difference in whether you actualize things or not: your Shopping Galaxy!

LAZY PLUS

> **Little drops of water . . . make the mighty ocean.**
> —JULIA A. CARNEY

This game is an easy one to do, but it requires you to connect with another person. This is CONSCIOUS SITUATION in action, showing how even a little bit of *raising the bar* can change everything! (This one requires no pregame warm-up, because it involves an event.)

THE SITUATION

Any casual, *in-person* event that includes you and at least one other person. For example, a simple coffee date with a friend.

THE TASK

Add one little extra to your regular casual, "lazy" outfit. For example, take your basic hang-about outfit and add a hat, a hair ornament, a bit of jewelry, a fun pair of shoes. You simply wear whatever you would to a casual meetup and add this ONE item. It's not about how "appropriate" this item is, it's just about the adding of one thing to a regular "lazy" outfit.

THE RESULT

After the event, record anything the addition influenced—the event itself, your friend, anyone else who might have been involved, your own experience.

EXAMPLE

THE SITUATION

I met up with a friend to have a little catch-up for coffee and gossip at our neighborhood outdoor café. As this is a super-casual place, and it was a mild spring afternoon, I simply wore a sweater over leggings, my usual throw-it-on-and-run-out-the-door outfit.

THE TASK

I added a little hat I picked up at a thrift shop a few months ago because it tickled me. This was a vintage "Juliet cap" with a flower appliqué. It was a lark purchase, and I never had the chance to actually wear it before.

THE RESULT

We had a lot of giggles about my hat, which created a lighthearted atmosphere. Also, several women stopped to comment on how they loved the hat. The energy was definitely uplifted by this one little plus. We actually had more fun than we have had in a long time!

RECORD YOUR LAZY PLUS BELOW

THE SITUATION

_____

_____

_____

_____

_____

_____

THE RESULT

_____

_____

_____

_____

_____

_____

THE TASK

_____

_____

_____

_____

_____

_____

Now that you've gotten a taste of how even a dollop of CONSCIOUS SITUATION can change the outcome of your EXPERIENCE, let's move up a bit in the aspiration department. We are going to explore how this can give you results that are more far-reaching in your life. Your dreams are about to drop in for a visit!

DREAM JOB/DREAM EVENT

> *The surest way to make your dreams come true is to live them.*
>
> —ROY T. BENNETT

What I'm going to ask you to do now is to connect your present situation with your dreams. This game is also designed to show you how your passion ALWAYS connects with your higher purpose. I want you to experience the POWER your style has to make your dreams come true.

Start this one with your pregame warm-up so you can get centered to help you envision your dream job. It will take you right to the one your heart desires.

1) Go to zero. 2) Pull up your awe. 3) Do Susan's Breath.

STEP ONE: VISUALIZE YOUR DREAM JOB. (DON'T BE LIMITED HERE. THE ONLY CRITERION IS THAT IT STEMS FROM YOUR PASSION.)

THE SITUATION: You have a meeting with someone IMPORTANT connected to your job. And this meeting is vital to your success in this job. This means this meeting will require an upgrade from your normal everyday work attire.

YOUR UPGRADE: What do you put together to make this impression count and help you advance? The only requirements are you have to make it specific, and you have to go all out in creating an HTT that will help you nail your dream. (You have no limitations, such as in budget, etc., as this is a dream after all!)

HERE'S AN EXAMPLE: JOSIE

DREAM JOB

BIRD VETERINARIAN is Josie's dream job. Her usual work attire is scrubs.

DREAM EVENT

A fundraising cocktail party with potential backers for her potential bird hospital. She has to upgrade from her everyday scrubs to make sure these benefactors will take her seriously as a stellar candidate for sheltering their substantial investment.

HER UPGRADE

Wanting to walk a delicate balance between dressing up and still appearing serious, she opts for a two-piece silk shantung suit in forest green, with a marigold silk blouse. She picks up the green in elegant pumps and carries a marigold/green combination in a leather clutch. Simple gold earrings and a gold brooch complete her HTT. Her hair has been twisted into a refined updo held in place with a tortoiseshell comb.

She has kept herself relatively conservative but is still dressy enough for a cocktail party. This helps her project the level of upscale yet not ostentatious presentation that is serious enough to allow her backers to feel comfortable with her. It's the polish without flash that her HTT captures that is crucial for nailing the financing of her dream. This is the POWER OF HER STYLE in action!

All you need to do is let your dreams lead you to play this game. You don't even need to be in the job market to do this. Maybe you're retired. Possibly you are a stay-at-home mom.

Just go to the place of "If I had the opportunity to land the dream I've secretly harbored, how would I navigate this game?" It does not require any part of your current life's situations.

This game is designed as an important step leading toward our upcoming shopping section. Playing it will release you from constraints that hold you in place instead of allowing you to fly forward. I am going to help you learn that successful shopping cannot be separated from your dreams! So, play this game with all your heart. Remember that passion is the direct link to your higher purpose.

RECORD YOUR EXPERIENCE HERE

YOUR DREAM JOB

_____

_____

_____

YOUR DREAM UPGRADE

_____

_____

_____

YOUR DREAM EVENT

_____

_____

_____

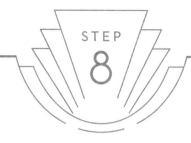

YOUR GALAXY
OF DREAMS

SHOPPING!

If it's not in your closet, it can't be in your life.

We've spent so much time during our journey uncovering all the amazing parts of what nature has blessed you with, but none of it matters if we can't also get it into your life! It's such a simple premise, yet it is the one that trips nearly everyone up at some point.

If you want to truly come into your own Authentic Style, you've got to have the clothes! And where do we get the clothes? *The store that sells them!*

How do we accomplish this? We change everything about HOW YOU SHOP!

Shopping should be fun, but it also should be effective. This is where there tends to be a vast disconnect in what most often occurs in the store.

We all shop with different motivations ruling what we actually buy. The one that invariably gets left out at the checkout counter is the most important: YOUR POSSIBILITIES.

The most common problem is: Most of us have huge holes in our closet when it comes to what is possible!

Your closet is the place that should connect where you are today with where you want to be tomorrow.

The awesome power of shopping is that it offers you the tangible bridge between your dreams and your "reality." This bridge is your version of a painter's tools. The clothing and accessories you procure at the shop are just as essential to manifesting your style as Monet's paints and brushes were to composing his *Water Lilies*.

So let me help you assemble your own "paints and brushes" in the way that will turn your shopping experience into *the place where magic happens*!

When Susan and I are at the point where we are shopping for clients, the organization is critical to making the experience into a victorious one. (We will have previously put the client through the transformative workshop where we have already completed all the analysis and education necessary as well as have begun the transformation.)

So at this point, if you were our client, we'd assemble all your pertinent information. We'd have your Season and Image Identity and all your sizes at our fingertips. We'd have also asked for your work information (including current and dream jobs) and a dream board, in which you would have previously created for us composed of all sorts of images including clothing as well as other things that inspire you. (These can come from art, nature, architecture, etc.—anything that makes your heart sing.) And last, we'd have a budget.

This gives us all the information we need to get into the store and pull the outfits that will cover the range of possibilities for the client. (And this can range from one outfit to an entire extensive wardrobe.)

Now, since you are DIY-ing, you will have amassed a version of what Susan and I do as our necessary preamble to shopping simply from playing all the games that have led up to this point.

THREE KEYS TO VICTORIOUS SHOPPING

1. **HAVE A PLAN**

2. **SHOP BY OUTFITS** (no unrelated separates)

3. **SHOP-PORTUNITY!** (Shop with an open mind)

Let's go over these points in brief before we continue.

HAVE A PLAN. What are you looking for? An outfit for a specific event? A new wardrobe? Replenishment/updating your existing wardrobe? Write this down on paper (or record on your phone) and DO NOT GO INTO THE STORE WITHOUT THIS PLAN. While this one may seem obvious, it's the major factor in why those impulse purchases keep your credit card company thriving while your wardrobe pays the price! Think of your plan as your best friend who is keeping you from embarking on the *Titanic*!

SHOP BY OUTFIT. Remember you are ALWAYS making HTTs, whatever the situation, from work, to casual, to special occasion. So you have to create them IN THE STORE. (I always say to everyone, "*The store is where the transformation happens!*") This means you SHOP BY OUTFIT, one outfit at a time.

Shopping for unrelated separates is a surefire wardrobe killer! You cannot get close to achieving your style with a bunch of separates that don't connect. Even for the most casual situations, you need to be *creating an outfit*. Shopping piecemeal can be a hard habit to break, but it is critical. Be ruthless in changing this practice. Also, don't leave the store with an incomplete outfit. I can promise it will hang in your closet like a sad jilted lover!

SHOP-PORTUNITY! This one is going to stretch you at first, but it will be the most fun in the end. Remember playing Potluck and Don't Fence Me In? Now's the time to refresh your memory about the things you preconceive (such as "I have to have waist emphasis") and your prejudices ("Mustard makes me look like a hot dog!").

Don't cheat yourself out of new things you aren't used to. Each shopping event should be a TREASURE HUNT. Mine the racks for the gold hiding in between the yucks!

Each trip should be a DISCOVERY of new ideas. Today, stores turn over complete inventory like mad! There are so many fabulous new designs that you can integrate if you remember what you've learned via your games. It's a new day of fabulous color possibilities and unexpected fabrics. EXPECT THE UNEXPECTED!

EACH SHOPPING EVENT IS A TREASURE HUNT!

LET'S PLAY MAKE-BELIEVE

A VIGNETTE OF SHOP-PORTUNITY IN ACTION

I want you to pretend you are a fly on the wall with me as we explore how this mining for the unexpected works. Let's visualize how this might unfold in one specific outfit in a make-believe situation.

Let's imagine a dear friend of yours has a new job interview she really wants to nail, an executive position at a media company. She knows she needs something very professional and polished but also sophisticated and current. It's an investment purchase, so she's given herself a budget that is on the high end of what she is willing to spend. *Remember, this position is one she really desires.* (This is also a great example of the Dream Job/Dream Event game coming into a real-life scenario.)

Now let's go through the mechanics of what could happen once she is in the store. She's got her PLAN handy, right where it can keep her in line. She's on the hunt for the gold.

As a Dramatic-Classic Bright Winter (size 8 on top, 10 on bottom), she has in mind a stylish, upscale suit. At the shop, she goes over to her size on the rack. She sees several tailored jackets (most suits today are sold as separate pieces) in deep colors that seem possible. She finds a lovely one in a deep wine and tries it on. It looks right, but just as she starts hunting for the coordinated slacks, she spots a very elegant wool crepe dress in a gorgeous purple with wide navy satin banding at the collar and hem. It's so captivating, she decides to give it a chance. Voilà!! It's perfect! While the wine suit was very good, this dress is a knockout, while also perfectly fulfilling all her requirements. Totally professional yet totally chic and sophisticated. Your friend's style in spades!

Now her task becomes to turn this stunning stand-alone into a showstopper of an HTT. Moving to the shoe and accessory area, she finds a per-fect pair of deep-purple suede pumps, along with a navy leather clutch with purple edging. Next, she unearths an earring that is a navy enamel crescent that up-curves on the ear, while at the same time also creates a repetition of the sleek updo hairstyle she's already got in mind.

So to recap, this is what your friend did: She had the plan. She kept an open mind (that's how she ended up with the perfect dress instead of the "good" suit). By adding the perfect accessories, she then elevated a simple dress into a showstopping HTT that would give her a leg up in her job interview. *This is shop-portunity in glorious action.* It's how the unexpected became a life-changing treasure!

Now, this could just as easily translate to a neighborhood barbecue for which your friend procured something along the lines of a fun toreadors/print top outfit capped off with a little shrug and finished with sandals, hoops, and a twisted head tie.

Or your friend could be shopping exactly the same way for a wardrobe, as long as she does it *one complete outfit at a time.*

Speaking of wardrobes, it's a good idea now to talk about what is the ultimate goal in terms of building a fabulous and successful one.

First, remember you always have two simultaneous goals. Number one is to have every outfit be as special as you are! From the most casual knockabout to the fanciest evening and every situation in between, you want to always rock your Season and Image Identity!

The other thing that I want you to experience is what I call *the jumping-out-of-bed effect*! I want your entire wardrobe to delight you to the point where each day you can't wait to get dressed! If you don't have clothes that make you want to leap from your bed into them in the morning, then you are missing out!

It's just as easy to get dressed in the best outfit as it is in a mediocre one, *if you have the right ones in your closet*!

So now we have an ultimate goal of a wardrobe of nothing but outfits that are A1, blue-ribbon winners! The key then becomes: How do you get there?

There are several different wardrobe plans that can take you from wherever you are today to that place where your closet is complete. Let me give you a couple of the best ones I've created over the years.

Assemble a calendar where you have room to write out a complete HTT for each day (either on your phone or on paper). Your task is to fill in either one or two weeks of HTTs, with each day outlining a completely separate outfit. What I want you to do here is take your calendar from BLANK to BRIMMING, one day at a time!

Now of course, you have to make a budget. (I'm going to help you with that in just a bit. For our current purpose, we are going to simply assume it's adequate to fulfill what I'm outlining below.)

Entering the store with your plan, you start shopping for each day. You have a SITUATION FOR EACH DAY PLANNED, BUT NOT AN ACTUAL OUTFIT. Let's say you know Monday is an office day, Tuesday is a Zoom-meeting-at-home day, and Wednesday is an errand day, but also you have a casual standing lunch with a friend, and so on and so forth.

Now you have determined three days of HTT NEEDS, and you can begin your hunt! Don't "pre-insist" on something. KEEP AN OPEN MIND. Your goal here is to find the hidden treasure, the gem you didn't even know was there!

Here are examples of what three days could look like on your calendar. (And remember, HTT means you always include ALL accessories.) For our purposes now, I'm using the Winter palette.

MONDAY (work in office)	TUESDAY (Zoom at home)	WEDNESDAY (errands plus casual lunch)
Royal blue blazer	White silk blouse	Hot pink/white cotton sweater
Royal blue slacks	Fuchsia blouse	White capri pants
White silk blouse	Fuchsia/blue print silk scarf	White sandals
Navy pumps	Navy leggings	White straw bag
Navy bag	Fuchsia enamel earring	Pink hoops (earrings)
Silver circle (with pearl) earring		White Bakelite bracelet
		White/pink straw hat

After you have completed your calendar, go back and add at least one "extra," which we will call your UNEXPECTED DELIGHT. The only requirement for this is that it be something out of the ordinary. Go back to one of the games that took your dreams into consideration. Make sure this one is elevated from your everyday life. (A good choice is often something dressier than you are used to, but it doesn't have to be.) This falls under the *wardrobing your future* department. Don't shortchange yourself out of this one. It could be the one that changes your life!

Now, I realize, of course, everyone can't start by shopping for a complete week or more's worth of clothes at a time. These are PLANS you start shopping with. Whatever funds or availability you have, start DAY BY DAY.

ONE DAY'S CONSUMMATE HTT IS WORTH A KING'S RANSOM OF RANDOM SEPARATES.

You may be thinking this is going to require a huge wardrobe with so many different pieces it is out of reach, in terms of both volume and finances. NOT SO!

This is where the beauty of this new approach comes in. One of the reasons I created this method that combines both style items and color palette is to make it within everyone's reach! (Listen, I live in a city where closet space alone is more valuable than a penthouse!)

Your Season is a family of interrelated colors, and your Image Identity is a group of interrelated styles. Your PALETTE and your PERSONAL LINE give you a built-in coordination. Once you start shopping by HTT, using your Season and your Image Identity as your guides, along with your plan, you will actually have fewer clothes.

It's the *shopping by separates* that gives you the overflowing closet with no successful outfits.

What you want instead is *a closet that opens to reveal a perfectly curated collection of HTTs that fulfills all of your situation needs.*

Fast-forward in your mind to the time and place where you have that blue-ribbon wardrobe where everything hanging in your closet is your personal best. The colors splay out like an array of your personal rainbow, and all your outfits hang side by side in perfect harmony. You have amassed all the accessories providing the finesse for every HTT.

You have truly built a complete wardrobe that fulfills your current life and also is a stepping stone to your future.

At this point you have a different set of needs when you shop. Your basics are covered; they just need periodic updating. Twice a year, in the spring and the fall, you can make a trip to the store to tweak things. A *refreshment* of your closet.

This is important, for even though your styles have a timeless basis, everyone needs to stay in touch with the changing mores. Your closet needs to keep evolving as you evolve.

However, at this point you are beyond the overhaul that being beholden to trends requires. At the same time, if you find a trend that you really would like to explore, you can afford an outfit or two that allows you that foray into a lighthearted bit of gratification.

It's important to remember that "timeless" doesn't mean "dated," just as sure as "trendy" doesn't mean "modern."

A curated closet keeps your style rooted, so you can keep moving forward without losing your identity.

QUIXOTIC SURPRISES

The supplemental things that can occur at this point are PURE FUN—what I call *shopping for added attractions*. This is when you are in the phase of *augmentation and expansion*.

For instance, since you already have the shoes you need for every HTT, you can pick up that extra pair that shouts out to you. The extra little bags, the fun jewelry—this is when you have the chance to succumb to accessory heaven.

Whereas before your wardrobe was a curated collection of HTTs, you had to make sure which didn't include accessory holes, now you can throw caution to the wind! (If your heart desires, of course.)

Now, of course, you are still staying within the parameters of your Season and Image Identity. That should be considered simply a given at this point in your journey. These supplements are your closet's equivalents of "cherries on top of your sundaes." They are wardrobe "top-offs" that are only relevant when you have the basic "fixins" underneath settled in.

ONE DAY'S CONSUMMATE HTT IS WORTH A KING'S RANSOM OF SEPARATES!

TIME TO START THE QUEST

Now it's time to venture into the store, where your dreams hang on the racks (side by side with a few nightmares!), just waiting for you to claim your future. Let's get you ready for a fabulous and fruitful treasure hunt!

Shopping itself is a loaded event for most women. Even if you are the type that views shopping as your recreation, there is a way to approach it that will give you a better experience.

For many of us, shopping carries with it a lot of baggage. (And it's the baggage being brought into the store I'm speaking of here, not the kind you are leaving laden with!)

Shopping has the potential to be an experience of total delight. There's magic at your disposal when you know how to conjure it up. On the other hand, it also can be a place where the dark forces of insatiable commerce and confusions collide!

So, the first thing is to prepare for the battle.

By that I mean simply realize that there are lots of minefields in every store. While some of these may indeed be in your head, some are actual danger zones that are built into the stores themselves. (The draconian dressing rooms, for instance, which we are definitely going to tackle here!)

Let's assume you've got your plan in hand, and all the things we've previously discussed are all in place for your campaign.

The first thing to do in preparation is DRESS TO IMPRESS—YOURSELF! Don't underestimate the value in looking your best to shop. You're going to be staring at yourself in a distorted mirror in horrible lighting at some point. If you start with sloppy clothes, messy hair, and little or no makeup, you're entering the arena with a big handicap.

I'm not suggesting you need to pull out the hats and gloves from yesteryear here. I'm just saying dress like you are looking forward to a day of fun rather than it's no different from doing the laundry!

By the way, if you are disposed to shop with a friend, be very selective about which one! Sometimes your best friend is your worst shopping companion! Choose wisely, using your history as your selector.

It's attitude, not aptitude, that's the goal here. By that I mean a friend who's less of a fashionista and more of a *loving heart* is going to be the most valuable helpmate for you.

It's the support, not the critique, that will help you when you get into the dressing area.

At this point, you are entering with your own new sense of color and style that you've painstakingly gained. You really don't need (or want) strong opinions that aren't centered in what you've found out for yourself.

What will help you most is the friend who is your *confidence builder*. That's the one inestimable quality that I suggest you make sure any shopping buddy passes muster for.

BEFORE YOU DIP YOUR TOES IN THE WATER

The first step in achieving VICTORY THROUGH SHOPPING occurs before you set foot in the store. No matter whether you are shopping for one outfit or a complete closet transformation: Stop off somewhere—a little café or a lunch counter, for instance—and *enjoy a pre-store treat*. Go have coffee, sit for a moment, and just catch your breath. Give yourself a bit of delight, collect your thoughts, and allow yourself a peaceful beginning. Refer back to your PRE-GAME WARM-UP here: 1) Go to zero. 2) Pull up your awe. 3) Do Susan's Breath.

It's really, REALLY important to start with a positive and hopeful frame of mind *before you even set foot in the store! A bit of bliss will set the mood for a fabulous excursion!*

Now let's move through the doors and onto the floors! Let me take you by the hand and let's go shopping together!

MINING FOR YOUR DIAMONDS IN THE ROUGH

> *It's hard to be a diamond in a rhinestone world.*
> —DOLLY PARTON

I've shopped all over the world, in stores from New York to London, Paris to Tokyo, and everywhere in between. Whether it's Madison Avenue or Rodeo Drive; from Ginza to the Champs-Elysées; down to the Fast Fashion Emporium and the Bargain Barn—I always start with the same two-part technique.

PROCESS OF ELIMINATION; GATHERING POSSIBILITIES

The fuller the stock in the store, the more digging through excess you have to do. The only way to weed through the abundance of merchandise is to *get rid of the surplus first, so you can start creating from the "possibles."*

This is where knowing your Season and Image Identity really proves their value. Since you know your colors and your style range, why waste time with things that don't fit within your parameters? Get rid of these fakers that lead you astray—those rhinestones that clutter your vision and leave you confused—and you will leave yourself *the pile of your diamonds in the rough*!

Out of this group you will discover things that will be unexpected dazzlers. Things you couldn't have even imagined as possible before you uncovered them.

So don't ever again spend hours combing through tons of items crammed together on the rack. Don't ever again go into a store hunting for a preconceived little black dress that doesn't exist. Don't ever again leave empty-handed after hours of fruitless scouring, lamenting, "They didn't have a thing in that store for me!" (Truth be told, they did! You just passed them by!)

My experience has proven that to almost invariably be false. The problem isn't the lack of appropriate stock, it's the way we traditionally shop. There is almost always something fabulous just waiting for you to uncover it!

From now on, enter with your battle plan, stick to it, and save yourself time, energy, and money and leave with genuine, bona fide diamonds!

FOLLOW THESE SIMPLE INSTRUCTIONS FOR A FAIL-SAFE SPREE.

1. Go to your size on the rack.

2. Eliminate all colors not in your palette. (Keep EVERYTHING in your palette.)

3. Eliminate all styles that are obviously not in your range.

4. Then, without any judgment, take what's left into the dressing room and try them each on. (By "without any judgment," I mean don't decide whether you like something or not until you've tried it on.)

This is where you will find the unexpected diamond that was waiting for you!

Next stop—the dressing room! (Ye gods!!)

FROM ALCATRAZ TO WONDERLAND

RECLAIMING THE DRESSING ROOM!

> *Become the sky. Take an ax to the prison wall.*
> —RUMI

Whoever designed the original dressing room found in the women's department must be the same man (and it couldn't have been a woman!) who designed the first prison colony!

You think I'm joking? Well picture this: You are locked in a windowless cubicle. Its temperature is set to basic meat-locker freezing. Overhead the fluorescence turns your skin to a shade of pistachio only a Martian could love, while speakers set at an ear-splitting volume keep relentlessly pounding disco pumped into your cell. As the pièce de résistance, you are required to face yourself in various states of undress in front of a warped fun house mirror! This is *la chambre minuscule* where you are asked to max out your credit card!

Well, this is only a bit of exaggeration, but you get the picture. Remember when I brought up the concept of the two types of baggage you have to confront in the store? (The kind that arrives with you in your head, and also the kind that the store has built into everyone's experience there.) The dressing area is where they collide. So let's tackle this obstacle and shed some much-needed light and love into this space so magic can happen there!

(This is going to occur after you have amassed *your haul of possibilities* and are ready to bring them to the dressing room for your eagerly anticipated try-ons.)

At this point, we want to go back to game number one and expand it to . . .

MY THREE LOVES (DRESSING ROOM VERSION)

The first thing to do is start with a positive mindset. After arranging your haul, take a moment and go back to your pregame warm-up: 1) Go to zero. 2) Pull up your awe. 3) Do Susan's Breath. Take as much time with this as you need. Don't be intimidated by thinking you have to rush. This is your time in the dressing room. *You have every right to spend as much time there as you feel is necessary.*

Next, take a moment and look at your three loves from our very first game. (I hope you recorded them both in the book and also on paper.) Let them sink in.

Now, take the note and tape or stick it right on the mirror. That's correct, *I want you to be able to include your three loves in your line of sight when you are looking at yourself in your try-ons.*

As you slip into each new garment, keep breathing, and keep your "awe" image in your head, right with you. If you ever feel yourself slipping into a critical mode, stop yourself, go back to your warm-up, and take the time to repeat the three steps.

You may need to practice this before it becomes second nature in your dressing room experience. It does take time to overcome being captive to the *dressing room blues.*

Now, I realize everyone has a different history here. But whether the experience has been traumatic or just uncomfortable for you, these rooms are the "black holes" of shopping where all the things you've been brainwashed with seem to crash together.

REDECORATE!

> *Some people look for a beautiful place, others make a place beautiful.*
> —HAZRAT INAYAT KHAN

You have the power to change this space. When I say it is the place where the magic can happen, I'm not speaking metaphorically. Your dressing room is your potential CHAMBER OF TRANSFORMATION.

It's important to remember that while the store controls the outer parameters of this room, you have the power to turn the inside of it into a warm, supportive environment. Anything you bring with you that helps you stay rooted in your heart is worth bringing into this space.

Earbuds playing soothing music can make a huge difference. (A little Mozart, for instance, can go a long way in helping you stay in touch with a higher beauty.)

Sometimes bringing in a *transitional object* can also help. We have a client who always pulls out a little marble heart from her purse whenever she tries on clothes. She told us her favorite aunt gave it to her when she was a child and she was going away to camp to embrace whenever she felt homesick. She told us throughout her life, this little heart had carried her through all her scariest moments. (Boy, did that bring up some waterworks from Susan and me!)

Make it your task to do anything that will help you turn your dressing room experience from a torture chamber into your personal wonderland. It should be the cocoon that allows your transformation, so that each time you step out in your try-on, it's like the emergence of the glorious monarch you are!

Now let's move on to a thorny subject, but one that has to be addressed and reworked for you to get to the checkout counter with the ultimate swag for your style to come to fruition.

YOUR BUDGET

> *Don't be a martyr to your imagination.*
> —SHERIDAN HAY

One of the biggest roadblocks to breaking out of your style rut and capturing your dreams is the lack of imagination when it comes to budget.

Now, let me reassure you that I am very conscious of responsible planning when it comes to shopping. In fact, I am pretty famous for being a budget whiz when it comes to creating wardrobes.

Susan and I work with budgets in all ranges, from the smallest to the largest and everything in between. Over the years, I have shopped couture, and I have shopped bargain basement. I have also heard every excuse in the book about money and lack thereof.

It's NEVER the money that is the issue. It's always the client's commitment to investing in herself, OR her lack of willingness to do so.

I am not talking about extravagance as your ticket here. I am talking about not cheating yourself out of your birthright!

Being home-based in New York, one of the concentrated demographics among my clients over the years has been aspiring actresses. Agents and managers have sent me young women just as they are beginning to climb the ladder professionally for decades.

Now, if you've heard legends about starving actors, let me assure you they are all true! Actors, at the beginning of their pilgrimage, come to New York with nothing much except their dreams, a suitcase, and an empty bank account! Truly, these young artists often can barely scrape two nickels together, let alone contemplate financing their career needs.

Yet, because they have a commitment to their dream that is unwavering, they manage to come up with enough funds to invest in the necessary tools for them to maneuver through the business.

I especially love working with these young hopefuls, because they have the imagination to think outside the box. I don't care if someone comes to me with just enough money to obtain the bare minimum in an outfit. If they have the desire and the dedication, we can always find a way. It's about the creativity involved and the commitment to their dreams that allows us to succeed in our quest.

You have every right to make your dreams come true. You only need to be as serious about achieving that as you are about anything else in your life.

Susan always counsels the client, as they are making a budget to shop, to remember *they are investing in themselves*. She reminds them that they will invest in a house, a car, a washing machine, a partner, their children, even their cats and dogs—anything under the sun—but they don't put themselves on that list of what matters.

I have to admit, every time I hear that last phrase, it breaks my heart. And yet, it is so often the case. YOU MATTER! YOUR DREAMS MATTER! YOUR PURPOSE MATTERS! If only I could help you understand that investing in yourself is not only appropriate, it is vital to everyone you love. When you are at your fullest, the world around you rejoices. Everyone gains when you are your utmost self!

Now, I can't tell you how much you should put aside for this part of your journey. I can only encourage you to take your needs in this area as seriously as anything else in your life.

Put yourself first, and the rest will unfold. You are not meant to sacrifice your dreams or your purpose. That is why you came to this planet, after all. Don't fall for the false premise of *the nobility of deprivation*.

I will repeat, the issue is NEVER about the money. It's ALWAYS about the commitment to investing in oneself.

IT'S NEVER ABOUT THE MONEY— YOUR DREAMS MATTER!

REALIGN YOUR GOALS

WISHES FIRST, MONEY AFTER

Here's my suggestion: Make a goal for what you want to achieve. (This is, of course, a basic piece of your shopping plan, which we've already discussed.)

DON'T START WITH THE MONEY. That is a guarantee your shopping will be a big flop! When you start by putting a limit on your dreams, what you have done is imprison them in a tightly locked box. Dreams and wishes need air to breathe, room to roam, and space to ascend. Dreams need the freedom to soar, so you never want to contain them by putting a lid on them.

Start by what you WISH would occur from your shopping event. (It's just a wish at this point. This is your INSPIRATION. The sky should be the only limit to your wishes.)

Next, decide what you think you can reasonably afford to spend, and then increase it by 10 percent. This will get your juices flowing and stir up the proper energy so the shopping gods can start working in your favor.

Yes, there are indeed shopping gods, and when you alert them with your proper attitude, they start arranging things for you before you even set foot in the store. (You don't believe me? Well, you'll just have to wait and see, then!)

In all seriousness, if you make the inner commitment to investing in yourself, the rest will unfold. You will be amazed at how making this change in your attitude creates incredibly beautiful results! This is, after all, the exchange of energy we spoke about earlier.

In the words of the lyricist and novelist Paulo Coelho: *"When you want something, all the universe conspires in helping you to achieve it."*

Bearing this in mind, we are going to now play a game that will help you learn to match the energy of your dreams!

DON'T PUT A LID ON YOUR DREAMS!

DESERVIN' THE DRESS!

> *If you are not willing to risk the unusual, you will have to settle for the ordinary.*
>
> —JIM ROHN

This one gives you the chance to make a large withdrawal from *the bank account in the sky with the unlimited balance!* (Whatever you take out is immediately replaced times two, forever and eternally.)

Your Task: to pick the most fabulous outfit you can find for an extra-special event. **Your Budget:** unlimited, BUT with a MINIMUM of $5,000 for the basic piece. (And this does not include any accessories.)

You are REQUIRED to spend this $5,000 amount for this piece. NO EXCEPTIONS.

NOW: Before you do anything else, record your immediate reaction to these instructions. No judgment, just be honest. Here are a couple of possibilities: Indignation. Giddiness. Anger. Embarrassment. Sadness. It doesn't matter what it is, just write down whatever you instantly felt upon reading the required price.

RECORD YOUR ONE-WORD REACTION HERE:

_____

We will come back and consider your response in a moment. For now, continuing the game, I want you to start the hunt online.

FIRST: What is the event you are searching for? (It can be anything from a black-tie gala to an outdoor party, to a business event. It does need to be somewhere that you would want to be at your most dazzling. It doesn't have to be ultra fancy, but it does need to be important to you.)

Record the event here. (Describe it in some detail. Don't just give it a name.)

_____

_____

_____

_____

Now start the search. Online (or in magazines if you prefer), find the outfit that is going to be your showstopper. Go to sites that include prices. Search high-end designers, luxury department stores. Especially seek out places you never thought of going before. As soon as you do this, post it in your online scrapbook and record the link below.

Remember, this is a fantasy game. The sky's the limit. I'm not asking you to lay down a credit card here! It's all from that unlimited, automatically replenishing bank account you have in the sky!

You don't even need to find the accessories here; this is about the one base item of your outfit.

RECORD THE LINK FOR AND DESCRIPTION OF YOUR OUTFIT HERE (INCLUDE THE PRICE):

_____

_____

_____

_____

BRAVO! In completing this game, you've expanded your horizons by going outside what is likely your normal comfort zone.

Anytime you go from *what is* into *what could be,* you allow yourself to evolve. And, as we recall one of the earliest tenets of this NEW VISION of beauty is: **STYLE EVOLVES FROM IDENTITY.**

It's giving yourself the full *permission to evolve* that is vital to this part of our journey.

Therefore, what I want us to do at this point is to go back and explore that immediate reaction you had to this game, specifically to the price requirement.

Let's first make the commitment here to remember there is NO JUDGMENT for whatever word you chose to describe your reaction. Whether it ranged from shock to outrage, delight to giddiness or even to embarrassment, there is *no value pronouncement* to your first instantaneous response. Our purpose right now is just to IDENTIFY your reaction.

The reason this connects to your shopping experience is ultimately about finding out where you might have entitlement issues that hold you back from realizing your dreams.

This is, after all, a **FANTASY** game. There is no actual emptying of the wallet here! This is not the same as the games that were about manifesting your dreams.

There is a vast difference between our **FANTASIES** and our **DREAMS.**

Dreams are aspirations; I like to call them "carrots," the things we look to that inspire us to actualize happenings in our lives. It's not that they have to arrive true in literal form; rather, they lead us to create things our soul is longing to bring into reality.

Fantasies, on the other hand, are escape oriented. I like to call them *mini-vacations.* They give us a chance to go beyond anything we might actually manifest but allow us breathers to travel into visionary worlds.

Both are key elements of our human existence and vital for our happiness. But for this game, it's the imagination part that we are concerned with, as I have designed this game with two purposes for you to achieve.

1. To give your CREATIVITY full flight WITHOUT LIMITS.

2. To help you identify any emotional limits you bring to the table. (Shades of our Potluck game!)

The question really to answer after this game is not about how fabulous your sky's-the-limit outfit was; it's really: *What is the level of your* ENTITLEMENT *to the best life has to offer?*

I want to repeat here, it's never about how much money you spend, or, conversely, how frugal you are. It's about having the full ability to be able to fulfill your dreams, whatever they are. So any reaction that suggests you might have an issue here is worth noting. I don't want that to stop you when you are in the process of making them happen!

You know, often when Susan and I have a client in the store, we will get to the final haul, where we make the actual purchasing decisions, and fear sets in. It will cause the client to reject an item that she clearly would love to have and that in truth would have a minor effect on her budget. It's more of a *mental state* than a reality.

Invariably, the client will call us in about a week after her time with us, during which she has had the chance to let her transformation sink in, and literally beg us to go back to the shop and retrieve the rejected item. And it'll be long since gone!

Do you DESERVE THE DRESS? Well, yes you do! And if you have a hold on believing this to be true in this area, I guarantee it will keep a lid on your dreams.

OUR DREAMS LEAD US TO CREATE THINGS OUR SOUL IS LONGING TO BRING INTO REALITY!

YOUR WARDROBE CABOOSE

ACCESSORIES!

> *Accessories are the exclamation point of a woman's outfit.*
> —MICHAEL KORS

The reason we call them accessories is that they are designed to *accessorize an outfit*. This means they are the finishes, not the main events. Shoes, jewelry, purses, hats, coats—anything that is not part of the basic outfit needs to be chosen *after the fact*.

Remember that you are always seen in real life in a LONG SHOT. Social media often obfuscates this. But think about the LONG SHOT as anything that is visible to someone as you enter a room. This should be considered as PART OF YOUR OUTFIT. Many a spectacular HTT has been ruined by a choice of unfortunate footwear!

Accessories don't exist in a vacuum. You need to think of them as completing a theme. You know that feeling of putting that last piece of a jigsaw puzzle in place? That magical moment when the picture finally materializes? That is exactly the effect the relevant accessories have on the outfit they complete!

HARMONY. COHESIVENESS. COORDINATION. COMPLETION. These are your bywords for choosing the accessories that will make your HTTs sparkle.

The great thing about this system is that these things automatically go together when you know your SEASON and your IMAGE IDENTITY. You don't need thousands of pairs of shoes to go with every outfit in your wardrobe. You will find, once you have curated your closet, that there is a large crossover of accessory items.

On the other hand, at this point, you get to fine-tune accessories. Now is when you can be specific and go for the accents that thrill you. Once you have everything in place, it's all about the JOY factor.

ACCESSORIES DON'T EXIST IN A VACUUM!

DANGER ZONE! ENTER AT YOUR OWN RISK!

ONLINE SHOPPING

So far, all our shopping techniques have been geared toward in-store shopping. Today, we all do a significant amount of buying online. This is a very difficult area to navigate because you just don't know what you are going to get. I would be remiss if I didn't give you a bit of acknowledgment that this is a fact of our modern life that isn't going anywhere.

However, that doesn't make it easy, or even that effective. It's more about avoiding online pitfalls.

How many times have you ordered that fabulous cranberry dress, only to open a box filled with a bright orange monstrosity?

And let's not even get to the size part of your order. Sometimes you must wonder if they really did think your size 10 is the same as their size 0!

My only advice for online shopping is to be sure you have easy returns available. I know the convenience of online shopping is seductive. However, don't trust color presentation as accurate. Don't believe sizes are standard. Don't assume a photo of the style represents what it will actually look like. In fact, the best things to remember are:

1. **Don't assume anything.**

2. **Make sure the site offers easy returns.**

The best thing you can do is to save up for an in-store excursion for your major wardrobe purchases and do your fill-ins online.

If you belong to online fashion groups, often you can consult the "hive mind" to find out which specific stores are the most accurate and which are most likely to disappoint. I know the members of many of these groups are eager to give this type of help.

I'm not suggesting you never shop online. Just remember that what is being presented is not what is necessarily going to appear at your doorstep.

TIME TO BRING YOUR PURCHASES TO THE REGISTER!

To shop victoriously is to treat yourself with the dignity, the respect, and the self-awareness of your purpose on this planet. It is the place where adventure and excitement merge with the manifestation of your dreams. The store is the magical land where your possibilities become your reality!

Without this thoughtful, planned, entitled approach to shopping, all the efforts you put into dis-covering your STYLE elements are simply parlor games.

As we prepare to leave our shopping port of call to move on to our next destination, I want to leave you with the thought with which I began this leg of our trip:

If it's not in your closet, it CAN'T be in your life.

VICTORY IS YOURS!!

YOU CAME, YOU PLAYED, YOU CONQUERED!

CONGRATULATIONS! You've now finished all the games and you've won the prize *just in the playing of them.* The games have accomplished their raison d'être in our journey and now it's time to move on to the home stretch.

They will always be here to refresh, repeat, or just refer to as you feel the inclination.

What they have given you is the AUTHENTICITY OF YOUR EXPERIENCE, which is the one true link to your AUTHENTIC STYLE.

They have offered you a path that is reliably steadfast in veracity, never skewed by whims, trends, dictates, or others' opinions. No one can ever quibble with your EXPERIENCE, because it is yours and yours alone!

This is exactly the crux of what a DIY approach is all about.

You no longer have to rely on myths, misinformation, or the fallacy of ineffective quizzes and faulty typing.

By first *Embracing Your Subjectivity,* the games have vaulted you into the realm of *Intelligent Subjectivity,* which is allowing you to move forward with accuracy and confidence in ways they provide the sole access to.

Most important, they also provided you with the tools that linked your INNER and OUTER selves, which is your ultimate goal.

You will be amazed at how different aspects of their effect will keep cropping up, offering you new and fresh insights as your style continues to evolve.

What I want you to do now, however, is celebrate the efforts you put in. I also want to thank you for playing the games with me. I'm aware that it took a bit of a leap of faith to approach things this way.

While the games are truly gifts that keep on giving, you had to be willing to receive them. This is the greatest victory I could have wished for you. Because as I said earlier:

It's not that you have *to change, it's that you must be* willing *to change.*

That you were, and that you did—bravo, bravissimo! Now let's move onward and upward!

THE AUTHENTICITY OF YOUR EXPERIENCE—YOUR LINK TO YOUR AUTHENTIC STYLE!

YOU CAME,
YOU PLAYED,
YOU CONQUERED!

NOW LET'S
MOVE ONWARD
AND UPWARD!

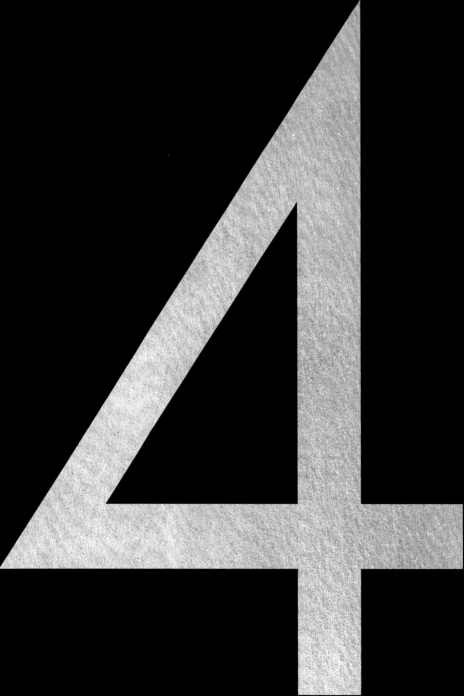

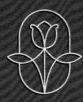

LOVE IS IN THE HAIR!

You only have one head; give it some glory.

As we move into the area that tops you off (your head!), I want us to go right back to one of the earliest images I gave you: *You are a PAINTING, and you are a SCULPTURE.*

Reminding you that this system I created is holistic, it stands to reason that for your hair to bequeath you its glory, it needs to be considered "one piece of the puzzle." It's not the most important piece, nor is it an inconsequential piece. Hair, like every other element of your appearance, requires *harmony* as its main goal.

Too often, women view their hair as a separate entity unto itself. That would be fine if you didn't have a body that your head is attached to! Much of the concern about and attention to hair (whether it be color or style) is traditionally connected too often to just the face. That might be fine if you were just a disembodied head, but *you are, indeed, a walking, talking, full-length, life-size human being*!

While it's true that your hair is a frame for your face, it is also the crest for your effigy! So let's explore how your hair can complete your entire persona most gloriously!

We know there are two parts to what your hair has to offer you: COLOR and STYLE. So let's approach them one by one.

COLOR YOUR HAIR (OR DON'T!)

> *Live beautifully, or dye trying.*
> —ANONYMOUS

> *I don't have gray hair; I have wisdom highlights.*
> —ANONYMOUS

To color or not to color, that is the question. Also, the answer! (By that I mean it's totally your choice!)

There is no reason that you should feel you HAVE to color your hair. There are many issues involved in making this decision. If you choose not to color, you don't need any advice. What's there is already a fait accompli.

On the other hand, there is no question that hair color, when done properly with the right goal and the right execution, can be a dazzling top-off to your appearance. (It can also be a disaster, but that's for later in our discussion!)

We've already broached your hair's color in our COLOR chapter (step six). So, let's refresh our memory about the way hair is (and must be) connected to your natural skin and eye color.

These three elements are a UNIT, paired together by both BASE (warm vs. cool) and DEPTH (clarity vs. dimension). They constitute a triad of genetically connected components, three interdependent elements created in harmony with each other. In other words, your hair color is never to be considered separately from your skin and eyes.

Your hair is ALWAYS going to be in the same family as your skin and eye color. There is never an exception to this. (Now, this isn't always so evident just looking at yourself. So don't get nervous if you don't feel you can see this yourself.)

Essentially, you want a *complementary frame for your painting.* That's the way nature created you. Therefore, that's our objective in how we want to approach enhancement.

Hair is the biggest block of color we see when we look at you. It's actually the biggest mass of color next to clothing that is visible when you are seen.

If you fight your natural coloring with an adverse hair color, it will do bad things to your face! It will create shadows, make your skin look sallow or faded, and make your face recede.

On the other hand, nothing can make your complexion glow, your eyes sparkle, and be the finishing touch that brings your entire being into glorious focus than a great hair color choice!

Once again: FOCUS is our holy grail.

The right hair color will focus you. The wrong hair color will make you fade away.

The two keys to choosing complementary hair color are the ones that your Season has already set out for us. (Bearing in mind that the way we determined your Season has already delineated what these two things are.) Base determines the family of your hair color. Depth determines the intensity of the shade.

Here's a chart of your hair color choices (and you can also refer back to the "Blueprint for Each Season" chart in the COLOR chapter for reference).

WINTER

*Color should be cool and vivid,
maintaining high or vivid contrast.*

Range: Black, cool browns (dark to medium dark), silver, white

Note: No warm tones, no red, no gold, no highlights

AUTUMN

*Color should be warm and rich.
Contrast level can be deep to medium.*

Range: Warm browns (from brunette to chestnut, from medium to light), all shades of auburn, deep tawny honey blond, warm gray, warm white; lowlights should be rich and multidimensional

Note: No cool tones, no highlights; color should not be light

SUMMER

*Color should be cool with subtle dimensions.
Contrast level is medium.*

Range: Cool browns (medium to light), cool blonds (deep to medium to pale), frosty gray, soft white; highlighting should be subtly dimensional

Note: No warm tones, no red, no gold

SPRING

*Color should be warm and clear. Contrast level
should be light/bright but not vivid.*

Range: Warm blonds (golden, yellow, honey), warm light golden brown, strawberry, clear red

Note: No cool tones; highlights should be light and bright, not too dark.

Two areas that often come up in terms of hair color are CONTRAST and DIMENSION.

Everyone needs contrast between hair and skin. There should never be a monochromatic level where the hair blends into the skin. That is the worst effect you can achieve in hair color. This is why hair color that is too light for a person's coloring is a disaster. It makes you look tired, washed out, and, let's be blunt: older in a not-attractive sense of the term!

Likewise, all hair color is technically dimensional. What that means is that hair up close is composed of different-colored individual strands.

However, what we are discussing here in hair color terms is EFFECT.

The effect of CONTRAST in hair color means a more solid appearance to the naked eye. The effect of dimensional in hair color is a more multi-toned effect to the naked eye. (This can be either rich or diffused.)

So, always remember when these terms are used in relation to the individual Seasons, it's the *effect* we are looking to create.

We are ALWAYS looking to use hair color in harmony with your natural balance of either warm or cool and either contrast or dimension. These are the guiding factors that determine the actual shades, including the allowable range from dark to light that will enhance and focus your coloring.

Now, in terms of communication with your hair colorist, they will have a different language. They use terms like "level," "red," "ash," and "neutrals," among others. This is different from the way we are learning them and the two languages should not be confused.

Hair color is a group of chemical products mixed together. Hair colorists think and work in accordance with this as their technique. As a layperson, it's best if you don't try to communicate that way.

You want to think in the terms that are outlined here in this book. Use them to communicate the EFFECT you want to achieve to your colorist. Let them translate into their chemical language to create the actual formula.

Our reasons and terms here are created for different purposes. (For instance, in formula terms, there are neutral colors. In your natural hair color, which we refer to in defining your Season, there is no such thing.) Don't get confused by this. Remember that chemicals require specific mixtures that are unique to their makeup.

If you choose to color, be prepared to take a little time to get used to the change. You've been looking at one person in the mirror for a long time. This new you is going to need a bit of LOVING introduction!

Hair color today is a miracle of modern chemistry! Done properly, it doesn't create the same "wear and tear" as it did in the old days! There is no question that a creative and complementary use of hair color can absolutely transform you! I love love love hair color as a choice for a dazzling effect that is YOU at your finest.

However, let me say again, there is never a need to color your hair. There are definitely times I don't recommend it. If you don't feel the inclination, then bless you and keep you! You are already a product of nature's best!

THE SHAPE OF THINGS TO COME

> *To sculpt a head of hair with scissors is an art form.*
> *It's in pursuit of art.*
>
> —VIDAL SASSOON

TIMELESS HAIR is the hair you want to achieve. It's your signature hair that will both evolve with you through time yet stay rooted in your AUTHENTIC STYLE.

I've spent many decades as both the owner of a salon that was a part of my studio, and also a trainer of both stylists and colorists from all over the globe. While new technology and advanced products are constantly being introduced, the principles of creating *timeless hair* remain the same. It's just a matter of helping everyone expand their techniques to include a broader vision of what each individual needs in achieving your ideal hair.

What SILHOUETTE is to clothing, SHAPE is to hair. The best approach to achieving what I call timeless hair is rooted in the *precision cutting technique* the groundbreaking hairstylist Vidal Sassoon made famous in the 1960s.

The concept pioneered by this hair revolutionary is often described as *architecture for the hair*. It's premised on creating a strong foundation for whatever the resulting effect might be.

The key to producing this structure is based on *cutting the shape into the hair*. Then any styling methods are considered the *finish* once this shape is firmly established.

Before I explain, let's distinguish and define a couple of terms we are going to be applying to our discussion here.

HAIRSTYLE refers to the result once all is said and done, including the cut, the finish, and any extra touches. It's the sum total of all the processes once everything is completed.

SHAPE is the outline of the hair. For it to be effective, it needs to be literally *cut into the hair*.

STYLING and FINISHING refer to the methods used to create the final result. This could include a blow dry, a hot roller set, curling irons, hand crimping, finger waving—anything you do after the cut that finalizes the actual hairstyle.

When you have a shape that has been cut into the hair, it does two important things that cannot be achieved any other way.

First, it allows your hair to fall into that shape. You don't have to manipulate your hair into it.

Second, it allows you to *connect your hair to the rest of your appearance*. The proper shape is a direct link to your proper silhouette. If we continue our analogy of you being a sculpture, then you must consider your hair as part of that sculpture. It's not something that occurs separately, pasted on top of you!

We will soon learn how when your shape and silhouette go hand in hand, you carry out the COHESIVENESS we have been seeking from the first steps on our journey! For your hair to be playing its part to perfection in your appearance, it needs to be considered one more piece of your puzzle.

On the other hand, when your hair and your clothing are disconnected from each other, you have that old hodgepodge that is the archnemesis of your forever goal: FOCUS!

A clean, defined SHAPE is the foundation that any great hairstyle must be built upon. The shape of your hairstyle could be considered akin to the structure of a building. The FINISH would then be the décor.

Without the shape being actually cut into the hair, you have to try to maneuver it into place.

Whether your end hairstyle is a smooth bob or a fancy, ornate face frame, the proper *precision blunt* cut is ALWAYS the base that you want to use as your foundation.

Once the shape is cut, then the styling and finishing can be applied.

HAIR TODAY—GONE TOMORROW

TIMELESS VS. TREND

> *Your hair is the crown you never take off!*
> —ANONYMOUS

Hair, like clothing, has cycles that can be rooted in timeless style or victims of capricious trend! The only difference is that hair trends take a lot longer to change than trends in clothes. So much so that the fact that they are, indeed, trends, and not "modern styles," gets overlooked.

When you look around you and see everyone having the same basic effect in their hair—that is a trend.

When you look at a person and the hair isn't a standalone that you notice apart from the overall STYLE of the person—that is MODERN.

Hair trends are manufactured "looks" created to sell images and products. You can see them often on the red carpet, or on celebrities in their personal appearances.

Timeless hair is like timeless style. It comes from your AUTHENTICITY and IDENTITY. While you certainly want your hair to evolve with the rest of your style (and your life!), you also don't want it to surrender to the crazy whims of trend that erase your individuality in pursuit of being like everyone else.

Hairstyles and colors definitely do need to change through time. There are many reasons for this. The good ones come from being in harmony with the actual evolving mores of society and your own evolution, as well as advances in technology that create new, exciting possibilities that previously didn't exist.

The not-so-good ones come from marketing sources that want you to blindly follow whatever is dictated as current hair fashion.

The problem with the latter is that, despite what is promoted, it's always a one-size-fits-all approach to hair.

If social media decrees a center part is de rigueur, then God forbid you show up with an off-center break! No matter that center parts create the most unflattering frame for your face, or that it might just ruin the overall effect of your personal style!

It's always disheartening to see celebrities show up on the red carpet in a $20,000 beaded gown topped off with a sloppy hairstyle, just because that's the current trend.

Timeless hair, on the other hand, allows you the freedom for both: It considers what's best for your style and also respects the situation as important factors.

Timeless hair allows you to update but not succumb!

YOUR HAIR AND YOUR IMAGE IDENTITY

I'm a queen, and my hair is my crown!
—ANONYMOUS

All you need to do to connect your hair to your Image Identity is to go back to your Yin/Yang Balance and your Personal Line. What SHAPE is going to be harmonious with your Balance?

Let's look at the extremes to get the concept.

EXTREME YANG (sharp, narrow): PERSONAL LINE: Vertical and narrow. Clothing style is sleek. So the shape of the haircut should have *a very defined outline* that is cut into the hair. This is in harmony with the rest of your appearance.

EXTREME YIN (soft): PERSONAL LINE: Curve plus double. Clothing style is soft and fluid with ornate detail. So the haircut should have *a curved outline with soft edges (which are finished)*.

Can you see the concept is simple? Connect the outline of the hair and the silhouette of the clothes. Once again, it's the COHESIVENESS of the HTT that counts.

Now, of course this is just general. There are numerous ways to create the actual hairstyles that are generated from the initial shape. The point is to start in HARMONY with what you've already discovered and connect your hair via a complementary SHAPE.

That's just step one. Of course, you also have to consider and respect the natural texture and makeup of your hair. For example, if you have thick, extra-curly hair, you can't expect it to lie smooth and flat in a sleek hairstyle.

Likewise, if you have very silky hair, you can't expect it to end up as a wild lion's mane!

You have to work with a great hairdresser to come up with the exact best hairstyle that combines both the CONCEPT and your individual hair. It's not one or the other. It's BOTH. But the big mistake that is often made is to ignore that you need to connect your hair to your overall STYLE first and foremost. Respecting the texture and growth pattern can still be achieved without sacrificing this.

Here's a rundown of each Image Identity and their respective hair needs.

To begin with, let's define two terms we will be using:

YANG CUT: *A strong blunt outline.* The edges are very defined. Sometimes there may be asymmetry along the edges or around the face.

YIN CUT: *A smooth-curved blunt outline.* The back is longer and then subtly curves upward. To achieve a face frame, there should be two slightly longer pieces next to the face on either side.

There are a myriad of ways to achieve these. To see some of these concepts executed, check out both the photos in "The Transformations" section, as well as the hairstyles on the ILLUSTRATIONS of each Image Identity.

YIN

SOFT DRAMATIC

Yin cut with a strong sweeping face frame.
Full and finished hair is required.

ROMANTIC

Yin cut with a soft face frame.
A finished look is required.

THEATRICAL ROMANTIC

Yin cut with a smooth and defined face frame.
Finished hair is required.

SOFT CLASSIC

Yin cut with a smooth face frame.
Finished hair is required.

SOFT NATURAL

Yin cut. A loose finish combined with a
smooth face frame.

YANG

DRAMATIC

Yang cut. The edges should be sharp and geometric.
Short to medium length but always very angular.

DRAMATIC CLASSIC

Yang cut with a smooth and angular edge.
Symmetry with an extra bit of sharpness.

FLAMBOYANT NATURAL

Yang cut. A strong outline with a
loose finish.

FLAMBOYANT GAMINE

Yang cut with asymmetry.
Short, face revealing.

SOFT GAMINE

Yang cut with a round outline.
Short, face revealing.

COMMUNICATING WITH YOUR HAIR ARTIST

Always be nice to the person holding scissors next to your head!

—ANONYMOUS

Hair is the one element of your appearance that truly requires an outside person having jurisdiction over what's going to face you in the mirror for at least a month!

Hair can be the most fraught area for many of us. Our hair is filled with history, dreams, regrets, pain, fear, and every emotion known to humankind! The fantasy of the perfect hairdo is almost mythological in intensity for so many of us!

Yet in the end, hair is just a stand-in for our deepest sense of self.

Yet it doesn't have to be the trial by fire we often make it! Really, a bit of common sense and another reminder to come from your heart will definitely go a long way in turning hair terror into hair delight!

Remember that your hair is a collaboration. You need to inspire and come from a place of cooperation. Too often, we approach our hair designers from a place of fear. Like everything else we've discussed, your goal should be to come from a place of love.

It's important to remember that people who have made a career of hair genuinely want to help you. They go into this field out of a love of beauty and a desire to share that with you.

They are also artists. Trained for years in their area of expertise, they have knowledge and technique that are at your disposal, if you learn *how to communicate with them.*

That being said, they all have different ways of practicing their art. They also have varying degrees of bedside manners. Your job, if you want to elicit the best of your hair person, is to learn how they work and do your best to be accommodating.

(On the other hand, if you run into the rare hairdresser who isn't interested in your well-being, absolutely find another who is!)

To recap: *Respect, but be clear. Listen, but don't ask for the impossible.*

Some hairdressers love you to bring in pictures. Some hate that. The biggest problem with pictures is the "unrealistic factor." You place your hairdresser in an untenable position if you bring in a photo of a style that is impossible for your hair type to achieve.

On the respect front, don't treat anyone at the salon as your personal lady's maid. Coming in with filthy hair is a big no-no! Put yourself in the shampoo person's position!

Also, if you show up to your appointment in a sloppy outfit and no makeup, with your hair a total wreck, you only make it that much harder for your stylist/colorist to give you your best effect.

One of the greatest ways to communicate with your hair person is to come to the salon decked out in a way that clearly suggests your STYLE. The visual statement you make in appearing this way can take the place of a thousand words of explanation.

It stands to reason that your hairdresser may need more information than the technical terms of your Season and your Image Identity, so give them visual cues to help them. Also remember it's the effect that is key. They will often have different terminology. Don't get hung up on that. Go over the charts for both your Season and your Image Identity. There are words there that will translate through all the different languages of the salon.

Also, don't put your entire sense of yourself in your hair! It's the finishing touch, not the golden fleece.

And most important of all, remember: HAIR COMES LAST. If you want to rock your personal TIMELESS HAIR, it's the crown you top your STYLE with.

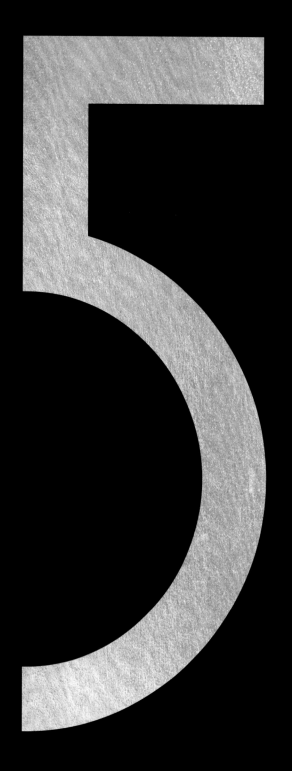

PART

5

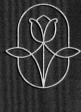

LET'S MAKEUP!

IT'S YOUR FACE. . . . WEAR IT WITH PRIDE

> *Beauty begins the moment you decide to be yourself.*
> —COCO CHANEL

> *The most beautiful makeup of a woman is passion. But cosmetics are easier to buy.*
> —YVES SAINT LAURENT

Our mythical belief in makeup as a tool of transformation has to be traced back to Cleopatra. She ruled an empire while rocking a wicked eyeliner!

In our modern time, we can trace makeup as it's known to us back to Max Factor. The foundation and blush you wear today go straight back to this cosmetics genius.

I've been developing my own unique approach to makeup for over four decades. In this time, I've consulted for both the largest of the global cosmetic brands as well as numerous smaller boutique labels. I've also created, revised, and refined my own makeup line for our private clients.

Most important, I've spent these years creating and developing my own techniques for the art of makeup and the way it fits into my overall philosophy of the why, how, and wherefore of what makeup can and should do!

As you can imagine, since Love-Based Beauty is holistic in nature, I have a very unique method of makeup that is going to be unlike any of the traditional directives you have ever been presented with.

Years ago, as a child, I remember watching the red carpet for the Oscars one season and being taken aback by what I was seeing. A cavalcade of women in glorious gowns that featured a lot of body skin were topped with faces that looked like they had been transplanted from someone else!

The suntanned arms, backs, and décolletages were plopped underneath pasty white faces with makeup so thick it reminded me of Kabuki! The disconnect was so striking, it stayed with me, and looking back, I can see where the seeds of what became my makeup technique sprang from.

What began then in the back of my mind was the absolute need to have a unique and foolproof system that connected the face with the rest of the person! This may seem obvious, but believe me, it is the opposite approach to how makeup has traditionally been presented.

Makeup still is taught as if it has nothing to do with clothes or hair. Yet who sees a disembodied face when you are out and about? No one, of course!

As my career progressed, I found that the products available in stores, as well as their basic purposes and applications, were simply not at all in line with what I was promoting. The colors, formulations, and application techniques were often actually in direct opposition to what I believed everyone needed to have access to.

Working first with my Seasonal requirements, and then advancing that to my Image Identity needs, I began what has become my own original design that not only revises the purpose of makeup but also gives you a one-of-a-kind, seamless connection between your makeup and clothing that is essential to modern daily wear.

This section of our journey will challenge many of the things you have been told about both what makeup is for, as well as how to use it. While you will want to start with a fresh perception, I can assure you the results will be well worth the willingness to revise your previous understanding.

Prepare to forget what you have been told, and open to a new idea that will allow your makeup to give you an entirely different effect and new sense of your true beauty! In the end, it's what's underneath that counts. I want to help you bring that out and merely refine and polish what is already there, so that your makeup is, first and foremost, SIMPLY YOU!

NAVIGATING SOCIAL MEDIA, TRENDS, "LIKES," AND PRODUCTS

Our current social media landscape has thousands of makeup tutorials offered at all levels of expertise, many of which are coming from teenagers. This isn't that surprising when you remember that the teen years are when most women start their initial love/hate/everything-in-between relationship with face paint!

The fact that makeup is readily available and relatively inexpensive coincides exactly with that point in life where young women are beginning to individuate and begin the steps on the lifelong journey of self-expression and the search for IDENTITY.

But just as we all evolve on our paths, so should the needs, reasons, and goals for using makeup. So perhaps we need to look at more sources than social media for makeup advice! While social media tutorials are often well-intentioned and definitely creative in their attempts, they are also wedded to the trends that we are seeking to go beyond in our journey here for the more timeless approach to your AUTHENTIC STYLE.

The most important thing to remember about makeup is that it's invariably connected to PRODUCTS. And wherever products are being used in your appearance, there are going to be companies that produce and sell them behind the scenes.

There's nothing wrong with this; it's a fact of life.

And as with everything else in the world, it's your EDUCATION that will lead you through the landscape of makeup products to discover *what actually works for you!*

Trends in makeup are like trends in everything else. *They are here today, gone tomorrow, and best taken with a big, huge grain of salt!*

Winged eyeliner, liquid liner, no liner, naked lips, frosted everything, Persian eyes, the no-makeup look, rouge, contouring, goth, glitter face, blue shadow, nude shadow, heavy brows, thin brows, no brows (!), thick base, no base—I could go on and on and on.

Whatever the latest trend in makeup is, you can bet your last dollar that tomorrow the opposite will be showing up on social media, along with the absolute admonishment that this is *today and the rest is passé!*

This is not going to change, and I'm not advocating for it to. Teenagers especially love to play with makeup, and they should!

On the other hand, I believe there is a much better, more sophisticated, and definitely more modern approach to makeup that you want to embrace as you get to the point where defining your AUTHENTIC STYLE comes into your life.

KEEP IT SIMPLE. KEEP IT REAL. ENHANCE, DON'T MASK.

There are no flaws, only unique characteristics.

My philosophy is to use makeup to make you look your best without calling attention to it. It should let your eyes sparkle, allow your skin to glow, and provide the finish and polish to your style.

What I am completely opposed to is the idea of "coverage" that creates a mask over the face!

Like everything else, when you start with self-acceptance, you end up with a radically different approach to makeup!

We have to start with this *philosophy,* because there needs to be a REASON for what you use makeup to do that defines everything else. This is what will help you avoid the traditional pitfalls, the false constraints, and a boatload of products that are not only unnecessary but actually detrimental!

WHY TRADITIONAL TECHNIQUES DON'T WORK

Traditional makeup techniques are always based on two things: *coverage* and *color.* Cover over your skin and paint a lot of color on top of that.

The biggest issue I have with this still-prevalent makeup technique (besides the crazy trends that can max out your credit cards and clutter your vanity drawer) is my much-hated archenemy: *the false idea that you have flaws that need correcting and covering up*!

When you start with that fake message, you are already doomed to be making a thick mask on top of your face. This "coverage" idea means layers of products overlaid on top of one another. The heavier the coverage, the more products you have to use overlaying them on your face.

However artfully done, this approach always ends up with an artificial mask that hides you. This creates a barrier between you and the world. It's tantamount to drawing a shade over your light!

On the other hand, when you have an approach to makeup that is based on ENHANCEMENT and FOCUS, you DEFINE yourself with a bit of makeup, properly chosen and applied.

ELIMINATING THE MASK OF "COVERAGE"!

ENHANCEMENT AND COORDINATION

Well, the great news is that 90 percent of your makeup needs are already met by simply understanding your Season. The remaining 10 percent is just the design of the products and learning some easy application techniques.

When all is said and done, and your colors are correct and you have practiced just a bit of brush technique, you should able to achieve the perfect makeup in five minutes!

For your makeup to work, the colors (eyes, cheeks, lips) have to do three things:

1. **BLEND INTO YOUR SKIN**

2. **BLEND INTO ONE ANOTHER**

3. **BLEND INTO YOUR CLOTHING COLORS**

Now let's examine the how and why these are requirements for your makeup to do its job. Remember that makeup is not solid color once it's applied. It's porous face paint. How it mixes with your skin tone is what matters, not how it appears in the container.

FIRST: *The colors have to blend into the skin to look natural.* This simply means warm skin tone requires warm makeup colors. Likewise, cool skin requires cool makeup colors. Your goal is for your makeup to blend into the skin, not sit on top of it, which allows your natural complexion to glow. Your Season automatically creates this.

SECOND: *You need to connect the colors of lips, blush, and eye shadows as a UNIT so they blend into one another and don't stick out individually.* You do this by coordinating both the FAMILY (warm or cool) and the INTENSITY (light, bright, or deep). The family is already established by your Season. The intensity is by design.

In short, if you are using a lighter lipstick, you also need a lighter blush and eye shadow combination. (Likewise with the brighter or deeper choices.)

Your goal, once again, is that three points on your face (eyes, lips, and cheeks) are balanced. From now on, NEVER think of a lipstick color by itself (or blush or eye shadow). It's the COMBO of lips, cheeks, and eyes that counts. (We will now refer to that combo as your *FACE*.) You are going to find you need *three Faces:* a *Light Face,* a *Bright Face,* and a *Deep Face* (all within your palette, of course).

THIRD: *At this point, you are going to need your Face to blend into your clothing colors.* Again, it's the FAMILY and INTENSITY match-up that will achieve this. (And again, your family is already automatically established via your Season.) Here's where you simply connect the intensity of your Face to the intensity of your clothing.

Each Season has three ranges of intensity for clothing colors within their respective palettes. In other words, you have your specific version of *"lights," "brights,"* and *"deeps"* for your clothes. So now that you have *three Faces,* you simply connect the intensity of your Face with the intensity of your clothing choice. (You will find the match-up of this on your chart.)

For example, let's say you are wearing a green dress. You aren't matching green to a specific makeup color. Rather, if it's a light green dress, you would use your Light Face. A bright green dress would go with your Bright Face, and a deep green dress with your Deep Face. It's NOT about matching *color to color;* it's matching *intensity of Face to intensity of clothing.*

This is the perfect way to use your makeup at its most effective: *using it as an accessory to your clothes.* Makeup as the perfect finish to your HTT. When your makeup blends into your clothes, you have the polish of finesse, the elegance of looking like your most focused self!

When your makeup fights with your clothes, you have either the clash of too much makeup or just the wishy-washiness of an incomplete look!

I realize that this is a lot of technical information and requires some fancy design ability in order to work. That's exactly why I created the three Faces technique.

By using the chart I am going to give you, you will have foolproof, automatic color coordination. Everything is BUILT IN! It will take all the guesswork, difficulty, and trial-and-error out of your daily makeup routine.

LEARNING YOUR ABCs

(You really did learn everything you needed in kindergarten.)

So you will now have three Faces, which I have labeled A, B, and C. Each Face goes with one of the three ranges of your clothing colors. (Each Face has a built-in connection of eyes, cheeks, and lips.)

Then I am giving you the specific RANGE within your palette that the particular Face blends into.

All you have to do is decide what clothing you are going to wear, and it will tell you which Face goes with that range.

At this point, *your makeup is truly an accessory to your clothes*. It's that simple and that foolproof.

Here is a breakdown of the individual colors of each Face and the range they go with:

ENHANCEMENT + COORDINATION = PERFECT MAKEUP!

KEY FOR EYES: **HL** (Highlighter) **OB** (Orbital) **LID** (Lid) **PEN** (Pencil)

WINTER

		A FACE: Brights	B FACE: Red/Deeps	C FACE: Pinks/Lights
LIP		Bright berry or magenta	Scarlet	Bright pink
BLUSH		Deep rose	Blue-red	Hot pink
EYES	HL	Orchid	Pearl, white	Lilac
EYES	OB	Royal purple	Cobalt	Mauve
EYES	LID	Plum	Navy	Heather
EYES	PEN	Dark plum	Black, navy	Grape

SUMMER

		A FACE: Pinks/Lights	B FACE: Reds/Deeps	C FACE: Purples/Brights
LIP		Rose pink	Raspberry red	Soft fuchsia
BLUSH		Soft pink	Rose red	Orchid
EYES	HL	Pink	Icy blue	Lavender
EYES	OB	Mauve	Periwinkle	Fuchsia
EYES	LID	Heather gray	Navy	Grape
EYES	PEN	Grape	Navy	Plum

AUTUMN

		A FACE: Lights	B FACE: Reds/Brights	C FACE: Browns/Deeps
LIP		Russet	Tomato	Copper
BLUSH		Deep peach	Bright brick	Bronze
EYES	HL	Goldenrod	Apricot	Tangerine
EYES	OB	Kiwi	Turquoise	Copper
EYES	LID	Olive	Teal	Sable
EYES	PEN	Forest	Dark teal	Espresso

SPRING

		A FACE: Pinks/Lights	B FACE: Reds/Brights	C FACE: Browns/Deeps
LIP		Coral pink	Poppy red	Bright peach
BLUSH		Geranium pink	Clear red	Apricot
EYES	HL	Apricot	Yellow	Gold
EYES	OB	Aqua	Jade	Honey
EYES	LID	Turquoise	Sage	Golden brown
EYES	PEN	Teal	Olive	Brown

SIMPLY YOU MAKEUP TECHNIQUE

(FIVE MINUTES AND BE DONE—BE GONE—BE YOU!)

Just like earlier in our journey ("That Was Then, This Is Now!" page 27), your face has to keep up with what's changed in our approach to the rest of your style.

The modern day needs a modern face, easy to apply and perfect in result! Simple, polished, and refined. *Makeup that puts* YOU *front and center* instead of showcasing gimmicky trends and over-done application.

There are two parts to my SIMPLY YOU makeup technique: *the color design* and *the application technique.* We've already tackled the former, so now let's get right to the fun part: *how to apply!*

First, I want to introduce you to the concept of a WATERCOLOR approach to your makeup.

This technique is based on the following:

1. THE COLOR DESIGN. All the colors blending together, and all the colors blending into the skin. *We've already accomplished this.*

2. CREATING A SOFT FOCUS WITH THE BLENDING TECHNIQUE. This means no sharp lines or defined outlines. This allows your features to be framed and put forward. (When you have defined outlines, your features recede, and the colors become dominant.) *This is created via your application.*

Once you practice this just a bit, you can literally accomplish the perfect makeup in five minutes. It's foolproof, easy to do, and will always give you exactly the ideal effect.

YOUR TOOLS OF THE TRADE: APPLICATORS, BRUSHES, AND PRODUCTS

Invest in a good set of brushes. Ninety percent of your technique comes from using a good-quality brush that is designed to create the specific effect. The rest is just learning to control the brush and blend a bit.

Brushes and Applicators you will need:

BRUSHES

Small concealer brush (thin)

Jumbo powder brush for overall translucent powder

Blush brush (smaller than the jumbo powder brush)

Eye shadow fluff brush (small with blunt edge)

Eye contouring brush (small with angled edge)

Eyeliner brush (small and thin)

Flat powder brush for blending (smaller than jumbo, with flat sides)

Brow and lash groomer brush, two sided (brush and comb)

Lip brush (small, tight, and thin)

APPLICATORS AND ACCESSORIES

Foundation sponge

Eye shadow sponge (for highlighter)

Pencil sharpener

Cotton swabs

Tissues

Makeup wipes

Small makeup mirror

Here's a rundown of the products you will need:

CONCEALER: Light, medium, or deep (*see color note*)

FOUNDATION: Sheer, water based (*see color note*)

TRANSLUCENT POWDER: Clear, colorless (*see color note*)

BLUSH: Three shades total (one for each of the three Faces)

EYE SHADOWS: Nine shades total (three for each of the three Faces)

EYE PENCIL: Three shades total (one for each of the three Faces)

BROW POWDER: (*see color note*)

BROW GEL: Clear

MASCARA: (*see color note*)

LIP PENCIL: Three shades total (one for each of the three Faces)

LIPSTICK: Three shades total (one for each of the three Faces)

LIP GLOSS: Clear

*CONCEALER: Choose a shade lighter than your dark undereye area.

*FOUNDATION: Choose a sheer, water-based product, either a warm or cool shade that ideally is slightly lighter than your skin above the jaw. (*With this type of makeup, you are* NOT *looking for the so-called exact match, because that will be too thick. You are looking simply to blend the tones in your skin with a bit of sheer, water-based foundation.*)

*TRANSLUCENT POWDER: If you have darker skin, choose two shades: one close to your foundation for the first step of application, and a clear shade for the second blending stage. If your skin is lighter, you use the clear shade for both steps.

*BROW POWDER: Choose a shade that is slightly darker than your hair color.

*MASCARA: Black for all Winters; black-brown for Vivid Autumns and Vivid Summers; brown for everyone else.

Now that you have the applicators and products assembled, we can learn this step-by-step application process. *It will be easy if you just follow the instructions and give yourself a few times to practice!*

NOTE: *The ease and perfection of results are based on all the products blending into one another. Don't make the mistake of thinking you can eliminate any of the steps. It's like the same jigsaw puzzle we've talked about previously. The picture is only completed when all the pieces fit together.*

APPLICATION TECHNIQUE STEP BY STEP: FIVE MINUTES TO *SIMPLY YOU!*

PREPARATION: Always start with a clean face. Any sunscreen and moisturizer needs to be applied and allowed to settle in for a few minutes before continuing.

CONCEALER TOOL: Concealer brush. Apply a small amount ONLY to dark area under eye with brush. Then pat into skin with fourth finger.

FOUNDATION TOOL: Foundation sponge. Apply a small amount (less than a dime) in various spots on the face, including eyelids. Blend INTO the skin with a damp sponge you have dipped in water. Foundation should not show up on skin. It should feel weightless on the face. DO NOT USE TOO MUCH.

TRANSLUCENT POWDER (FIRST COAT) TOOL: Jumbo powder brush. Dip one flat side into powder, shake off. Buff the face with a SMALL amount of powder. Be sure to include eyelids. Do NOT overpowder. This creates a matte finish and gives you the proper surface to blend the next colors into.

BLUSH TOOL: Blush brush. Dip into product. Crush color in palm of hand before applying on face. Apply UNDERNEATH cheekbone, starting at center of eye and sweeping upward into hairline. Take clean side and blend into skin. Think of blush as *shading*, NOT bright color for the cheeks.

EYE SHADOW (three steps)

1. **HIGHLIGHTER (HL) TOOL: EYE SHADOW SPONGE.** Dip into product and crush color in hand. Apply to entire upper eyelid, brow to lash line, corner to corner. Note: This is a sheer tint and provides the base color for the next two so they can be blended together.

2. **ORBITAL (OB) TOOL: FLUFF BRUSH.** Dip into product and crush color in hand. Apply to center of lid (on top of iris) and bring up slightly. It will appear as a soft smudge in the center of the eyelid. This color gives depth in the combination.

3. **LID (LID) TOOL: EYE CONTOUR BRUSH.** Dip into product and crush color in hand. First, apply to outer edge of eyelid, starting at corner and bringing in to meet the orbital color. Second, using edge of brush, connect the color from the outer edge to the brow bone. Then, *ON TOP OF BONE,* bring color inward about halfway. Note: This color should be applied on top of bone, NOT in the crease or underneath. This is going to be the frame for your eye. Follow the natural shape of the bone.

NOTE FOR EYE SHADOW: SEE DIAGRAM FOR EXACT PLACEMENT (HL, OB, LID)

EYE PENCIL TOOL: Eyeliner brush. Using colored pencil, lightly sketch a VERY SOFT line underneath and on top of lids. Start at outer corner of eye and go inward, about one-half to three-quarters of the way underneath the eye, and all the way corner to corner on top. Then, using the brush, smudge until line is erased. Your goal is a soft, smoky, thin smudge: a rim of smoke.

TRANSLUCENT POWDER (SECOND COAT) TOOL: Flat powder brush. Dip into powder. Shake off excess. Powder over blush to soften edges. Then do the same over upper eyelids in a horizontal motion back and forth until colors are blended together. Make sure outer edge is soft. This coat of powder does two things: blend the colors for a finished effect, and also sets the makeup.

EYEBROWS (THREE STEPS) TOOL: Groomer (brush side). Brush brows straight upward. Using the small stiff angle brush from product, dip into color and apply to brow until hairs are blended together. Then, using wand from product, apply clear gel to brow and brush upward. This seals the brow and sets color.

EYELASHES TOOL: Groomer (comb). Using wand from product, apply two coats. ONLY APPLY TO UPPER LASHES (not on bottom). Then, using comb side of groomer, separate lashes. Note: Don't overapply mascara. Lashes should be feathery, not thick and clumpy.

LIP PENCIL: Softly shade outer lip line. Keep on natural line. Do not go over the edge.

LIPSTICK TOOL: Lip brush. Dip in color. Paint lips until natural lip is thoroughly covered with opaque color. Blot with tissue.

LIP GLOSS DIP WAND IN PRODUCT AND COVER LIPSTICK. *USE MORE, NOT LESS! NOTE:* *You get a neat lip with the opaqueness of the color. You add a translucent surface with the gloss.*

NOW YOU ARE "SIMPLY YOU" GORGEOUS: GO FORTH IN ALL YOUR GLORY!

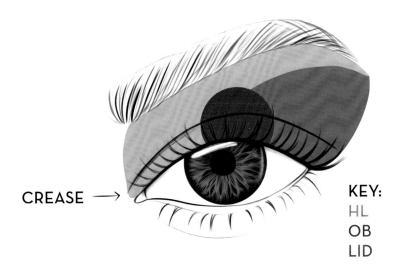

CREASE →

KEY:
HL
OB
LID

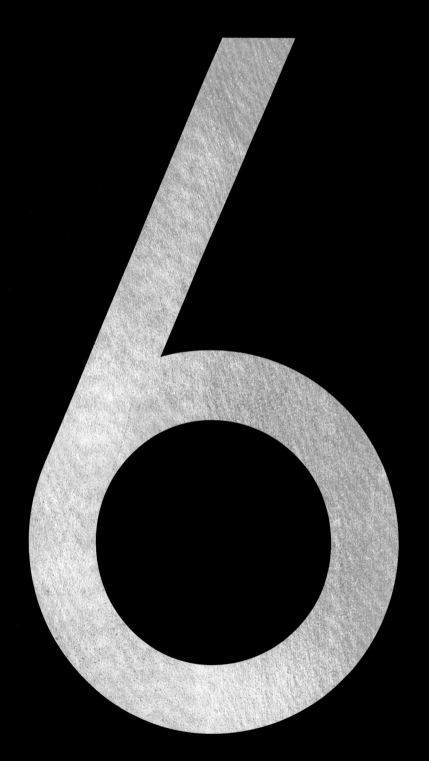

PART

6

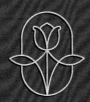

MYTHS, MISTAKES, AND MISDIRECTS
OF THE INTERNET

> *When you make a mistake, there are only three things you should ever do about it: admit it, learn from it, and don't repeat it.*
>
> —BEAR BRYANT

Ah, now we have to tackle social media and how it's been both a godsend and a devil's lair to Love-Based Beauty.

Let me preface this section by saying it is directed to those who have come into contact with these misdirects and been affected by them online. If you haven't come across them, feel free to skip over this and go merrily along to the next section!

For those of you who have been subjected to these, I realize you came to them in good faith. Misinformation is the big bug that infects the internet: *No one is making sure the information being spread is accurate.* Then, as incorrect information gets passed around, it gets farther from the truth, and the "new" version gets accepted as factual.

Sometimes I think parts of social media are like a viral game of GOSSIP:

Mrs. Smith has a new milkman servicing her today. Her nosy neighbor sees a strange man entering her house and phones her friend with the shocking news. By the end of the street, the telephone chain is reporting the sad news that Mrs. Smith has run off with a biker and is working as a stripper in Vegas! Her daughter Emily gets a text from her friend saying she is welcome to move in with her family.

On the one hand, I am grateful and delighted at the outreach that social media has provided. What has been a grassroots movement for decades has been propelled into the viral stratosphere by this engine of the digital age!

The flip side of this is the lack of oversight that has promoted major mistakes, misleads, misdirects, and outright falsehoods that send women on wild-goose chases and lead them directly AWAY from the desired results!

Everything that has come out of this new vision of Love-Based Beauty was created to give you your wings. To help everyone break free of the destructive dictates from the past that have kept you boxed into stereotypes.

Imagine my dismay when I see the information being perpetuated is a distortion of all that I designed, and the heartbreak I feel when I see directions and restrictions being attributed to my work that are exactly the OPPOSITE of all I set out to free you from!

So, what exactly have you been misled by? Why does it matter so much to correct this false information?

The primary thing that makes Love-Based Beauty unique is that it is HOLISTIC.

Since you are a whole person who was created to be uniquely YOU, so must your STYLE reflect you as that whole. All the old rules and approaches look at women as a bunch of individual body parts that need "correction" (or at least help) in order to achieve a false ideal. We've already gone into this at length, but how this relates to the misdirection of my work online is what we need to address if you want success.

It's not about whether someone has a different approach to my work or different opinion. It's about making sure that all the parts of what I've actually created are accurately presented so they can work for you. It also means eliminating the ones that are taking you in the opposite direction so they can be reversed.

At this point, let's simply identify and debunk these false directions so you can get the benefit of what I've actually designed. So let me list the major myths, misdirects, and misleads that are just flat-out wrong!

THE BIG THREE NO-NOS

1. **NO TYPING**

2. **NO REVERSE ENGINEERING**

3. **NO FAULTY ANALYSIS (AS OPPOSED TO DIY)**

Let me briefly explain what is being promoted that is wrong. (And by "wrong," I mean it's taking you in exactly the opposite direction of where you find your Image Identity and the freedom and empowerment that entails.)

MYTH #1

NO TYPING. The term "Kibbe Body Types" is a myth. Love-Based Beauty is about smashing the boxes of body types. "Body Types" start with a preconceived shape that you are then supposed to fit into. I completely reject that restrictive approach to style. IMAGE IDENTITY is the OPPOSITE OF TYPING!

The basis of Image Identity is better described as a sliding scale that puts YOU first. AFTER you discover the combination of your Yin/Yang Balance and your Personal Line, then, and only then, is the name of the appropriate Image Identity assigned. There are no types in my work.

When someone assigns you a body type, that's no different from the old and horrible fruit idea. How can you be an individual if you are a prune? You are a PERSON, not a TYPE!

"Typing" is short for "stereotyping." Anything preconceived is the OPPOSITE of my approach.

IMAGE IDENTITY is the name you give yourself at the END OF YOUR JOURNEY. There is no set style to your Image Identity. *It is a blueprint for your creativity and self-expression.* It's the visual "language" you use to tell your style story. *The story is YOU, not a preconceived label.*

I earlier described your Image Identity as your "style country." There are an infinite number of living places within your country.

Don't confuse your Image Identity with any preset style. It is your lodestar, not your destination. The way you express your Image Identity is determined by your taste, your situation, and your purpose.

By the same token, CLOTHES DO NOT HAVE IMAGE IDENTITIES. There is no such thing as "Soft Dramatic pants," for instance. The pants in an outfit for a Soft Dramatic are specific to that outfit. (See the chapters on PERSONAL LINE and SILHOUETTE, and the relevant games that lead up to them.)

The five ARCHETYPES *are symbols,* mythological in nature. They are just the general outlines that direct the beginnings of your journey.

The ten IMAGE IDENTITIES give you a focus that comes from all the things you discovered on your journey.

Instead of asking, "What's my type?," start by asking, *"How can I learn to see myself through loving eyes?"*

Then go to game number one: My Three Loves. That will kickstart your journey and set you down the path of self-discovery. This is the "land" where all the accurate answers are waiting for you!

Summing up, your IMAGE IDENTITY is the name that comes at the very end of the process. Take the journey and let it lead you to your Image Identity. Not the other way around. You have to start at the beginning, not try to jump to the end. There is no other way.

Which brings me to . . .

MYTH #2

NO REVERSE ENGINEERING. *You can't discover your Image Identity by backing into it.* It has nothing to do with the clothes you think you look good in. It's not about trying to identify body parts. Nor is it going to be found by staring at a photo of yourself.

Until you uncover your prejudices and preconceptions, your vision is skewed. What you are used to considering *good* is always subject to change. What you are "seeing" on a photo is simply not accurate. *What you are used to is not relevant to what you can be.*

Also, since clothes don't have Image Identities, what you think you look good in (or are positive you can't wear) has no bearing on what your Image Identity is or is not.

What you like is often not the same as what works. As you move through life, your likes will change, sometimes in the extreme. (I think back to some of my early likes with both humor and horror!)

Once you become proficient in the technique, then, of course, you want to love what you wear. But please, stay open to the new, the unexpected. (I refer you back to my "Holy guacamole" epiphany!)

STYLE is about discovering your POTENTIAL. Not what you are comfortable with or used to. You can't know what you need until you discover all the new visions of yourself. Otherwise, you are just repeating yourself.

It might be clothed in a new dress, but it's just a rework of the "same old same old." There's a whole new world of fabulous and new excitement waiting if you are simply willing to take a leap of faith!

There is no shortcut to style, because style is not something you see in a magazine, or on the red carpet. You can't quiz or type yourself to style. *Style EVOLVES as a result of the things that you EXPERIENCE along your journey.*

MYTH #3

FAULTY ANALYSIS (VS. DIY). *You CANNOT type others.* This is not possible and is a guarantee to a frantic and unrelenting spinning of the wheels—lots of effort that goes nowhere fast. As we just learned above, there is no typing of anyone. Nor can a group type others. That just compounds what was a faulty premise to begin with.

Analysis can only be done by a trained and certified professional. They have a very specific method of looking at someone that takes a completely different set of skills than anything presented in this book. This book is NOT a training manual for analyzing.

Whenever there is so-called typing online, it would be more accurately defined as faulty analysis.

What you CAN do is travel the journey of self-discovery that Love-Based Beauty is designed to

lead you on. This, as we learned in an earlier chapter, is called a DO-IT-YOURSELF (DIY) approach. That is exactly what this book lays out.

You undergo all the steps, and along the way, it's the discoveries and EXPERIENCES you undergo that lead you to the result. While you may not even realize it, just by playing the games, you change, both in vision and in perspective. It is sometimes subtle and sometimes more dramatic, but it cannot help but happen!

When you try to tell others what they are, you are only sharing what you see through the lens of your subjectivity (your prejudices and preconceptions). It doesn't matter whether you have a background or experience in art, anatomy, or even fashion; *unless you have the specific (and correct) training that a pro-*

fessional consultant has, you don't have the skill to be accurate.

One of the most important parts of the training for a consultant is the part that teaches them the safeguards that allow the circumvention of their personal prejudices. It is something that is very difficult to learn and takes a lot of time and effort, and not everyone can achieve it.

Now, most of the inaccuracies online are connected to those three major misleads. Here are a few others in brief, some of which we've touched upon earlier but need reiteration.

YOU CAN'T SEE YOUR PERSONAL LINE ON YOUR BODY. You can't find it in either a mirror or a photo. You have no "lines," and neither do your clothes. There is no such thing as "lines." I don't even know how that one got out, but it's dead wrong! PERSONAL LINE IS A TECHNIQUE. It is a connection between your body and a complementary silhouette. You have to SKETCH it according to the directions in the chapter that deals with this. There is no other way to achieve it.

Your body exists in three dimensions. Looking at it full front tells you nothing in relation to what clothing must allow. Clothing has to fit around all three dimensions, not just the flat surface you see in the mirror or in photos.

You don't see *width* on your body, for example. It only shows up when you have done the sketch that connects the proportions of your body as they relate to clothing needs.

Likewise, you don't see *Curve* or *Vertical* directly on your body. It's ALWAYS and ONLY visible ON THE SKETCH.

Of course, I realize this sounds complicated. That's why I created the technique of the line sketch that is foolproof and simple to follow.

But you must leave the false idea of looking for it on your body behind. It's not there. It's all about the sketch. It's a technique. The sketch is your blueprint. Not your body.

NO BODY PARTS. No *waist emphasis,* no accom-

modating *hips,* or *shoulders,* or *any specific body parts.* Your body parts are all INCLUDED in your line sketch. You do not single out individual parts.

Additionally, your waist is NOT a body part. It is the connecting point where your upper torso and lower body meet. It should be correctly referred to as your WAISTLINE. Therefore, there is no such thing as being *short-waisted* or *long-waisted.* This point of connection might be higher or lower on the body, but that would be totally dependent on *where the torso and lower part of your body meet.*

Similarly, having a natural indentation at the waistline occurs because of the curve in your PERSONAL LINE. For instance, a Double Curve will naturally come in at the midsection; it's a result of the curve.

The obsession with the waist is based on the old (ancient!) idealization of the forced hourglass silhouette that goes way back to the days of whalebones and corsets. If you try to force the waist into a silhouette that doesn't allow curve, it is tantamount to forcing a square peg into a round hole!

HONOR THE DESIGN INTEGRITY. Don't add a belt to a dress that doesn't allow for it in the design. Don't try to alter a silhouette with accessories.

Just because you CAN fit into something, it doesn't mean you should. This is an old sewing circle credo. It bears considering because social media promotes wearing clothing that is often too tight and too short. Don't confuse sexy with vulgar.

You don't have to be squeezed into a dress to look sexy! Body-con is a trend that is best worn in small doses. It rarely achieves the desired effect. You can look like a sausage if you force yourself into clothes that don't allow for your full self!

Details are subordinate to your SILHOUETTE and the DESIGN INTEGRITY OF THE GARMENT. There are no set necklines, skirt lengths, sleeves, or any other details of a garment or outfit for anyone.

Given the correct silhouette, there is no neckline that you cannot wear. (Likewise with any other detail.) How these things either fit into your silhouette or do not is the ONLY criterion.

A neckline never works (or doesn't) on its own. The design of the dress determines the neckline. The same with skirt length or type of sleeve. This is why you can't put a belt on a garment that isn't designed for it and expect it to work. *A dress that is designed as a column is totally destroyed by the addition of a belt.*

IMAGE IDENTITY IS NOT PERSONALITY. *Don't try to dress your essence and personality directly.* These will come out naturally after you learn the techniques of PERSONAL LINE and SILHOUETTE. Then, as you create an outfit via SITUATION, *your taste will allow these to emerge.* When you follow this system, they will all be natural outgrowths.

Personality and essence are subjective and ephemeral. *They are not things you can quantify.* They change according to the situation and others' subjective perceptions of you. That doesn't mean they don't exist. You simply don't want to force them. That leads to caricature.

Your face doesn't wear clothes. It expresses emotions. You don't dress them. You allow them. Your face doesn't need any clarification. Its beauty is clearly established. Makeup is the tool for enhancing its beauty. Clothes hang on the body.

Certainly, and emphatically, the basic premise of Love-Based Beauty is the INTEGRATION OF YOUR INNER AND OUTER SELVES. However, *this is an organic result of the technique when you follow it.* Of course, you want to express who you are on the inside through your outside. When you work in harmony with your painting and your sculpture, this naturally comes out, beautifully and uniquely, in the manner that is YOU AND ONLY YOU.

Once you learn the technique, it becomes all about your CHOICES. *Our choices become our personal statement to the world.*

RED FLAGS THAT NEED REWORKING OR YOU ARE SUNK BEFORE YOU'VE BEGUN!

Any comments that start with the following are a trap:

"I need . . ." (such as "I need to have a waist emphasis")

"I must have . . ."

"I don't . . ."

"I can't . . ."

"I know . . ."

Instead, I suggest you replace any statements that start with the above with:

"Let me *try* . . ."

Your style journey is about learning what you need, not what you are used to.

Be open to change. There are things you have yet to discover.

And always remember:

You don't *have* to change, but you must be willing to change.

IF YOU INSIST ON PRECONCEPTIONS, YOU ARE SENTENCED TO STAY RIGHT WHERE YOU HAVE ALWAYS BEEN AND CANCEL ANY POSSIBILITY OF MOVING FORWARD.

THE CELEBRITY TRAP VS. REPRESENTATION

> *In the future, everyone will be world-famous for fifteen minutes.*
>
> —ATTRIBUTED TO ANDY WARHOL

There is a reason I don't engage in the parlor game of celebrity typing. First, because typing, as I've emphatically made clear, is the opposite of what Image Identity is about. It's counter to everything I believe in and have based my work on.

I understand the desire to go down this road. But it's not only not helpful, it's actually detrimental in your own style journey. The main reason is: Especially online, people confuse celebrities with role models of representation.

Celebrities today are styled by celebrity stylists. The emphasis is on making a social media splash. The celebs also usually have endorsement deals with designers they are contractually obligated to wear in public appearances. This puts the focus on the clothes, not the person.

The red carpet used to be a cavalcade of stars. Now it's a lineup of designer endorsements.

Also, the information you can get online about a celebrity is faulty. Googled measurements have nothing to do with reality. Photos are distorted. So all the effort put into basing types on them is like a hamster's wheel of misinformation going round and round.

I want you to learn to look to yourself for your best inspiration. There is no celebrity who can ever be as marvelous as YOU! You don't want to borrow someone else's style. You want to claim your own style that is yours and only yours!

So just take all of the above with you as you travel the labyrinth of the internet and social media to help to avoid the pitfalls that take you off your path.

I don't want anyone who's fallen under the spells of these myths to feel uncomfortable or judged. I realize everyone is only searching for things that will help them in their style pursuit. At this point, however, it does need to become about accuracy and what will really help you. From now on, just look to this book as the source.

My clarification in identifying and debunking these myths is simply meant to keep anyone from falling into those traps.

I want you to succeed! That's my sole purpose.

THERE IS NO CELEBRITY AS MARVELOUS AS YOU— YOU ARE THE STAR OF YOUR LIFE!

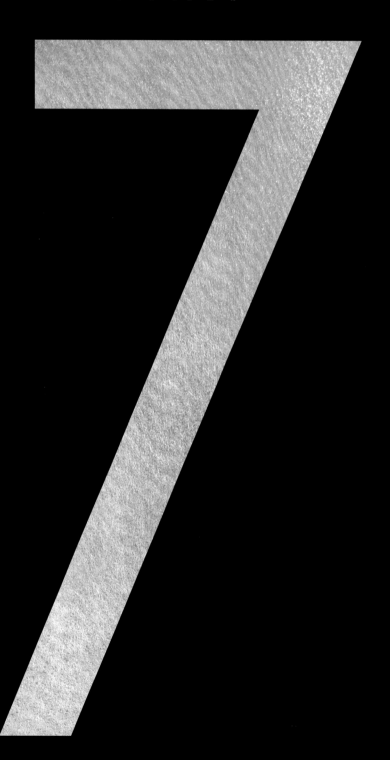

PART

7

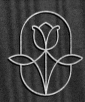

FROM MY PICTURE WINDOW

ON THE WORLD

PARTING REVERIES

I've been so fortunate to have spent my entire adult existence in the city I always felt would be my home. What I wanted more than anything else was to do something with my life that would leave the world better than when I found it! And I wanted to do that right where I landed, in the Big Apple!

New York is truly the destination of aspiration, the place that beckons to those who dare to dream as well as offers the possibility of making those dreams come true. It's the land where, whatever your background, race, creed, or sensibility, you can find a haven.

While it may seem overwhelming at first, it's really just a collection of small neighborhoods joined together that make up this giant metropolis—villages that jointly create this great melting pot of civilization.

My neighborhood is famous for being a place where all this diversity comes together. From my perch on a stool at the window of my favorite café, I get a front-row seat for the passing by of this gorgeous mosaic.

I often just sit and stare and contemplate. It's the perfect vantage from which to take the temperature of where we are now, as well as ruminate over things I've been lucky enough to discover in my time on this planet. It's also where I am continually able to evolve my theories, hone my techniques, and keep progressing.

From this viewpoint, I get the great opportunity to see what I feel is working and what needs to change. It's my "visual laboratory" and my intellectual workshop! So let me share some of the most important things I've learned that can help you as we wind down our journey.

THE PASSAGE OF TIME IS STYLE'S DESIGNER

AS TIME GROWS, SO GROWS OUR STYLE

Style and the passage of time are inextricably linked together. Their bond stems from both our brain's development as well as the evolving perception our experience provides us along the way. There is a natural development of what we learn style to mean and how it grows as we grow throughout our life.

In the beginning, most of us are dressed by our parents. We start our style journey in the complete control of the one who brought us into the world! This can be a great bonding experience or it can be a dictator/subject–type association!

I suppose I have a bit of a sense memory from the latter, as my sisters and I had a mother who thought of our dressing needs as photo ops! Oh, the uncomfortable outfits we were inserted into to get those "perfect shots of the perfect children" our mother lived for! It seems like I must have climbed out of the womb in itchy suits and bow ties, while my sisters somehow arrived in starchy petticoats. And don't get me started on our hairdos!

Somewhere along the way, maybe around five years, we begin to demand that our own voices start being heard. There is nothing quite as charming as seeing a six-year-old try to cram every print and color possible onto her tiny frame, and top it off with a tutu!

The *two Ts* define the era where our understanding of what we think of as style begins: TRENDS AND TEENAGERS!

The adolescent brain is defined as still developing through the early twenties. That is the time when individuation begins, while simultaneously is also paired with the need for peer acceptance.

In style terms, that means: rebellion! No teenager I've ever met wants to dress like their parents! (I know I sure didn't.)

I moved to New York when I was twenty. I had two approaches to style at that point on my journey. Because I was an actor auditioning for roles, I had professional needs. But in my private life, I was all about Fiorucci! (Look that one up for a real blast from the past.)

This is the stage of life when we need to experiment, as well as identify both with our peers and as a burgeoning actual person. It's about discovery, but still within the groups that replace our family units.

This time in our life means that trends appear as the style venue we relate to. Trends seem the ultimate goal for expression at this point. (And again, this connects directly to that "adolescent brain" stage of development.) And social media, with its *planned obsolescence,* is the perfect place for this obsession with trends to either flower or fester!

We've previously gone into the definition of trends, what creates them and the financial reasons that power them. No need to revisit that. Let's just realize that as important as trends are at this earlier stage in life, it's essential to move beyond them as we develop. If we hang on to trends as our guide for style, we become stuck in time.

I noticed at the very beginning of my work that the seriousness of purpose changed dramatically with clients at around the age of twenty-five. Life's needs changed, and so did their need to change how they both viewed and expressed their style. This is the natural time our style concepts will evolve, if we allow them to. Especially important in this time is to move out of the *"style is all about me"* attitude and into what I earlier called *sharing the sidewalk*. It's our connection to others that becomes our pathway to uncovering the true POWER OF OUR STYLE.

On the other hand, there is also a false narrative based on ageism we need to acknowledge and reject. This is the old poison that tells us at a certain point, we need to turn into our parents or our grandparents from an earlier era. That is just as destructive as hanging on to the false pursuit of youth with an iron grip that keeps us chained to our past while keeping our true potential left unrealized.

We should not succumb to the notion of fading away, just as we should not succumb to being a slave to trends.

All aging really is, is EVOLUTION. As time goes by, you are MORE of everything. You've learned more about yourself. You've gained experience. Instead of thinking that the bloom is off your rose, realize the truth that your beauty is *more full-blown*. So should your style be *more defined*. Each year, you get better. Until you decide to flee this coop we call Earth, let your blossoming continue! It becomes about SOPHISTICATION and RELATIONSHIPS!

RELATIONSHIPS ARE THE CORE OF YOUR ELEVATED STYLE

IT'S ALWAYS ABOUT THE GOLDEN RULE

> *If you contemplate the Golden Rule, it turns out to be an injunction to live by grace rather than by what you think other people deserve.*
>
> —DEEPAK CHOPRA

The last part of my window musings moves me to remember how relationships are vital to manifesting the true POWER OF OUR STYLE. In the end, at a certain point, it's the IMPACT that creates the greatest effect of our style as well as gives us the greatest JOY.

Remember at the very beginning of our journey when we were REDEFINING STYLE and learning about how it connects to our purpose? The NEW VISION OF LOVE-BASED BEAUTY? That style is the visual language we use to tell our story. And for our story to have any meaning, we need others to hear it.

When we move away from the narcissistic nature of our early days of style into a more enlightened state, we NEED to connect with others. That is where our true empowerment comes into play. *We want to affect the world around us.*

We may want to do that in either vivid and dramatic ways or subtle, quiet ones. But it always becomes about *sharing our energy with others.* What we put out comes back tenfold and then repeats. I think at our most exalted, style is really a CIRCLE OF LOVE.

This is where my thoughts go toward how we can do this in our modern world. We have so much fear and distrust surrounding us, especially online. Even in our online groups, there is a lot of negative energy, even vitriol, coming at us.

Well, this goes right back to the basic premise I started with. We have two choices in life: either to come from love, or to live in fear. I watch this play out every day from my perch at the window.

My own philosophy always goes back to what I learned before I can even tell you when: the Golden Rule (my version).

Treat others as you wish they would treat you.

Remember that you can make the world smile when you dress with your best self! There is nothing more fulfilling than knowing you've brightened the world by looking smashing.

Don't pooh-pooh that idea as superficial or silly. JOY *is the best energy you can spread.*

Doesn't it make you happy when you see someone walking down the street rocking fabulous colors?

You have no idea what thoughts you've inspired in someone when they encounter you at your most dazzling! Even little things can brighten the world around you.

Apart from all the techniques we've learned, in the end, you are a STAR, and the way you choose to lavish your light is your legacy.

When I stare out "my" window, I look for the best intentions of people. The little things. I don't look for what I think someone "should" or "could" do. I look for *what they are trying to do.*

Give a compliment when you notice an effort. It's not about so-called perfection. It's about the *aspiration.*

When you can't wait to get dressed in the morning because you love what you are going to be putting on, you've claimed your purpose. The rest will follow.

Look for the bliss that comes from sharing.

That's where you'll find your own Golden Rule applies.

Style, in the end, is about communication and connection. Love begets love. Approach your style this way. Be brave and share it with the world!

THE JOY OF SPECIAL

> *People of our time are losing the power of celebration.*
> —ABRAHAM JOSHUA HESCHEL

Before we finish, I have one last request. It's not really a game per se, but it is something you definitely need to actively do to benefit from its purpose.

Today, as has been noted over and over, we have become a very casual society. In many ways this has been an improvement over some of the rigidity that inhibited freedom in past times.

In other ways, however, I fear we have lost the power of celebration. And since this entire book is based on learning the techniques that releasing the true power of your style has the potential to achieve, then it would stand to reason that celebration is not just an important part of this journey, but it actually is also *integral to our fullest realization of it*!

To celebrate, we have to be making a statement that JOY is within our reach. We cannot celebrate unhappiness, or tragedy, or the blasé of daily routine!

As long as we are breathing and our hearts still beat, we can find things to celebrate! Life itself is a miracle, is it not?

Well, how about we take a moment to make time in our style journey to go beyond the casual of our everyday and bring SPECIAL into both our vocabulary and our life?

What I'd like you to do is pick a special place and dress like your life depends on it!

By this I mean go beyond your usual. If you normally go out to dinner in a super-casual way, pick a fancier place and dress up! Don't give in to the old "but nobody dresses that way here" adage. *Be the style leader of the pack!*

You will find you will be treated differently. (Better tables at a restaurant, for instance, will magically appear.) But more than that, you will bring JOY to whatever place you arrive at.

You will also discover the POWER that your style has to affect the atmosphere and the people around you.

And that, my friend, is the true POWER OF YOUR STYLE. As I said in the very beginning, style is how you share your energy with the world. Lavish your light on the world and you brighten it!

You have this POWER right at your fingertips any and every time you choose to call it up.

Give yourself the chance to experience the bliss that sharing your style with the world can offer you. THE JOY OF SPECIAL should be your everyday go-to!

With LOVE-BASED BEAUTY as your fuel and the POWER OF STYLE as your secret weapon, from now on, there's no more need to keep it such a secret!

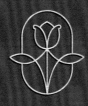

EPILOGUE

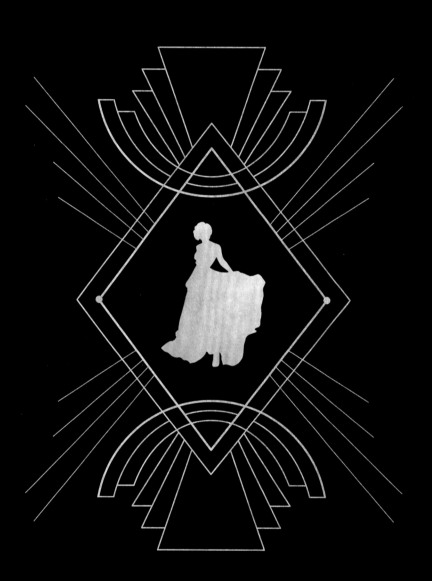

IT'S THAT TIME . . .

(BUT NOT FOREVER!)

> *If we can try with every day to make it better . . . the music never ends!*
>
> —ALAN AND MARILYN BERGMAN

Well, as we are coming to the end of our journey, we do have to say our goodbyes (at least for now).

My heart is full, but also tearful. I've loved guiding you on our trip, and what will I do now that we are parting?

I have tried to steer you on this path of self-discovery by sharing all the years of my experience. I've also put my heart and soul into every page of this book.

But what I also want to assure you is that as we come to a close, this isn't really the end.

Anytime you feel the need, have a question, or just want to touch base, all you have to do is open up this book and I am right there.

If there is one thing I want to leave you with (actually there are about a million things!), it's to repeat where we began all those chapters ago:

Style is a journey of self-discovery that evolves *from your IDENTITY. Since our identity is always expanding, then so must our style. It never should be set in stone or become static.*

That means we are always traveling this path together, because there is no limit to how far we humans can blossom! *We are always transforming into our greater selves.*

My most fervent wish has been to introduce you to this new vision of beauty, as well as give you the tools to release the power of your style.

At the same time, I hope our time together has been as much fun for you as it has for me! Because *if your Style is your superpower, then* JOY *is your rocket fuel.*

As we bid adieu, I want to send you off with love, with great appreciation for taking this trip with me and allowing me into your life. I am honored and humbled to have had you put your trust in me.

I wish you to always live beautifully, love beautifully, celebrate yourself, and to remember this:

The world is hungry for your light—GIVE GENEROUSLY!

I salute you as I bid you au revoir (until we meet again).

XOXO David

CODA

ACKNOWLEDGMENTS, GRATITUDE, AND CREDITS

As this book was decades in its appearance, it stands to reason that it could hardly be considered a solo effort. So many wonderful angels have helped me on my pathway to bring this to fruition, I want to pay tribute to those who have been instrumental in helping me bring this journey to you, so we could all travel it together.

SUSAN SLAVIN. By now you are aware that Susan is my wife, my soulmate, my muse, and my partner in eternity. What I also want to make sure everyone realizes is how essential her contribution here has been. I could not have asked for a better collaborator.

She has been with me every step of this process, from inception to completion. Down in the trenches with me every day, I could not have brought this work to the world without her involvement in every aspect, both in word and picture. The time and energy Susan devoted to helping bring this work to life is illustrative of her devotion and commitment to its message.

Every day I would come home from hours of writing and then read her my day's efforts. It was her stamp of approval for each portion that provided the impetus that kept me moving forward.

The photo shoot was a mammoth production, literally months in the making. Not only did Susan co-design every element of each model from hair to outfits, to makeup—she also produced the actual shoot itself.

The illustrations presented their own unique circumstances. Each of the thirty had the same artistic requirements and design by us as the live models did, yet it also needed the addition of the consummate artist who could execute our vision. After auditioning an endless number, we were at the point of having to revise our concept when miracle worker Susan found our *artiste supreme* on the other side of the world! With this factor involved, our need to navigate the extreme time change between New York and India found Susan communicating her revisions in the wee hours of the morning every day for six months. It is Susan's unparalleled eye for detail that made every illustration come to life.

Susan's heart and soul, her wisdom and artistry, is woven into the fabric of every page of this book. I couldn't have created it without her. She deserves more credit than I can give her, and my gratitude for her generosity and brilliance is boundless.

SUSAN

CREDITS FOR THE PHOTOS AND ILLUSTRATIONS

Each gave us the combination of their individual artistry, with the ability and grace to execute our design (no small thing with a system that is so specific as mine).

PHOTOGRAPHER: The incomparable Maurizio Bacci is *La Dolce Vita* materialized! He is the genius behind the camera, responsible for all the photos in the book, including the reveals, the front duo photo, and the back cover photo. Susan and I have worked with Maurizio for years. Every shoot is an artistic triumph and a celebration of life!

ILLUSTRATOR: Chandan Kumar Mohanty is the genius who hand painted each of our thirty examples in their finery, as well as did all the superb line drawings and other illustrations throughout the book. Besides being a brilliant artist, he is also the kindest and gentlest soul and a gem to work with. I've no doubt we will be hearing great things from this young man in the future!

HAIR TEAM: Brandi Veretto (color and style), Tanya Rullan, Melissa Pacheco, and Mirela Radoncic gave their all to execute Susan's and my designs in the glorious hair in the photos. They are each and every one darling and superbly talented women, and we love them all dearly!

MAKEUP: Don Rokiki added his beautiful artistry to execute my makeup technique. A master of his art and a delight all rolled in one fabulous package.

ASSISTANTS: Linda J. Calderon was the wonder woman who kept everything together. No detail too small, no request too large as she made sure things hummed along. Her fabulous daughter, AmyLinda Saez, stepped in during our second phase to provide the same essential production assistance. Both of these warriors kept chaos at bay in the most genial way. Lifesavers in action!

MODELS: These women all gave their own unique and special beauty to grace this book. It's no small thing to undergo the transformation process and endure the rigors of a shoot. I think they are all actually fairies, because they each appeared like magic for us! They are, in order of appearance: Melissa, Zyana, Rachael, Rivka, Brianna, Serena, Margaret, Paige, Angelisa, and Veronica. Volunteers all, special thanks is offered to these showstoppers.

JEWELRY: Katie Thompson (of KT Collections) was our fairy godmother. At a mere moment's notice, trays of her magnificent jewels would appear by special delivery. Generous to a fault and blessed with exquisite taste—she consistently saved the day!

If I could bottle the superstar that is my spectacular agent, Suzanne Gluck, I would be a billionaire (except I would want to keep the bubbling bottle all for myself)! Suzanne has it all at her fingertips. Smart as a whip while sparkling like a glass of vintage champagne, Suzanne has been with me from the beginning of time. She championed my first book and is the wizard behind this one. She is the best: best agent, best friend, and best lunch companion. Très brilliante!

To all my additional friends at WME: assistant Lane Kizziah, who looks like a Ralph Lauren model and functions like a CEO, Caitlin Mahony, and the "Ladies of the Book Nook." Special shout-out to Nina Landolo, who got things off to the greatest start during her tenure, as well as Tracey Thompson.

No book like this can reach an audience without an extraordinary publishing house and team. Rodale was perfection from top to bottom. My astute, patient, and gifted editor, Matthew Benjamin, both sought me out and shepherded me through the labyrinth of this process. He is a prince among men, for sure! Also, thanks to his great assistant, Mia Pulido, whose diligence and fine efforts are consistently the glue that holds things together. Paul Kepple for the stunning interior and cover design, Lynne Yeamans for her beautiful art direction, Jenny Davis (creative director), Robert Siek (production editor), Allie Fox (managing editor), Mark Maguire (production director), and Aja Pollack as copy editor all deserve great praise. I'd also especially like to thank Theresa Zoro (president) for including me in the Rodale pantheon, and Diana Baroni (publisher), who along with Matthew made the initial outreach that started the ball rolling. While I'm at it, let me just thank the entire company of Penguin Random House for being the home base of all things great and wonderful!

Very special thanks to three of my most special friends, my three amigos: Vanessa Prolow, Angèle Gautreaux, and Amy Turner, who have been my online guardian angels. They are three brilliant, loving, and gorgeous light bearers who created the basis of what has morphed into the viral "Kibbe World" on social media. Among their many efforts was the genesis of the Facebook group Strictly Kibbe. And speaking of that group, special love to the members who keep on growing so beautifully, day in and day out, and the moderators of all the sixteen groups whose volunteer efforts keep the fabulousness going and growing! Susan Friedl gets special thanks for being the queen of organizing transcripts. The brilliant and beautiful Chinu Ahmed deserves extra gratitude for her ever-ongoing graphic designs and inspiration. She is pure love and pure talent.

Thanks to Juliet, Loni, and Treany for being my entrees and gatekeepers of my beautiful office space at The Yard where this book emerged.

Great thanks go to the uber-glam Raquel Cabrera and all her merry band of baristas at my neighborhood Starbucks for creating the warm environment where I started each day's creations. They kept the iced tea flowing that powered my thoughts and dreams!

I have been so fortunate in my life to have had the love, support, and guidance from many wonderful sources. First is my beloved mentor, piano maestro, and soulmate, the late May Lindsay. So much of my artistic life is rooted in what she gifted me with.

The late, great Barbara Sher was another mentor and great friend whose wit and wisdom are a constant source of inspiration. My three celestial friends, Emmanuel, Abraham, and Julian, along with their earthly compatriots the late Pat Rodegast, Esther Hicks, and the late Rev. June K. Burke, are my loving conduits to the truth. I am so grateful to have been introduced to them long ago.

I am also thankful to my late parents for providing the pathway to my life and my two dear sisters who keep the family flame glowing. Big sis' Ann Kibbe, my party girl who never stops, and little sis' Jane Blank, my astonishing treasure. My late aunt Mary Hert, who growing up was a combination Auntie Mame and surrogate mom, introduced piano into our lives and brought joy to our hearts.

I'd especially like to give thanks and love to our "family of choice," Pamela Shaw and Victor Talbot. This couple has been with me from the very beginning, providing love and support every step of the way. They have been the touchstones of my adult life.

Lastly, I'd like to give great gratitude to all my wonderful clients who have traveled from all corners of the globe to work with me these last four decades. You have made my life an amazing adventure and have been my fabulous companions on *my* personal journey.

Onward and upward we go together as we fly to the sun and beyond!

xoxo
david

ABOUT THE AUTHOR

David Kibbe has been an internationally renowned beauty/style expert for over four decades.

As a top media personality, Kibbe has appeared on hundreds of TV and radio shows including *The Oprah Winfrey Show, Today, CBS This Morning, Good Morning America,* CNN, *Sally Jessy Raphael,* and PBS. He has been a recurring guest on Boston AM, as well as every major morning show in the country. With his upbeat message, he has also been a favorite of radio talk shows throughout the world.

In print, David has been the subject of countless features including *The Wall Street Journal, The New York Times,* the London *Times, USA Today, People, TV Guide, Allure, Harper's Bazaar, Glamour, Town & Country, Cosmopolitan, Ladies' Home Journal, Redbook, Good Housekeeping,* and *Woman's Day.* He was also the beauty editor for the syndicated magazine *Romance Today* (supplement to *Parade*).

Today he is profiled in a legion of online magazines, blogs, and podcasts, including *Vox, The New York Times, Bustle, Air Mail, Byrdie, Parade, Mel, Glam, The Sun,* and innumerable sites spreading his fame across every continent.

He is the creator of his celebrated "Head-to-Toe Transformation," wherein clients come from all over the globe to his New York City atelier for the chance to undergo "THE DK EXPERIENCE."

David's clientele, from celebrities to the average person, has also included major corporations such as Revlon; Estée Lauder; Avon; Johnson & Johnson; Procter & Gamble; Charles Jourdan; Bloomingdale's; JCPenney; Coppertone; Ballantine Books; Macmillan; Little, Brown and Company; JPMorgan Chase; Citibank; and Touche Ross.

His work has expanded into creating interior designs for clients, companies, and resorts in the United States, Europe, and Japan.

In his spare time, David has also created a thriving career as a triple-threat performer, appearing in original works produced by Lincoln Center, Neighborhood Playhouse, Primary Stages, Circle in the Square, Hudson Guild, and the Kennedy Center as well as having starred in two critically acclaimed one-man shows in New York City.

Previously, David authored the much-loved classic *David Kibbe's Metamorphosis.* Released in 1987, each subsequent generation since has kept rediscovering this groundbreaker, culminating in its current status as the continually recurring viral sensation of today's social media.

Rising above the present-day incessant turnover of fast fashion, and the constant mutation of trends, as *The New York Times* recently reported, Kibbe's work has "stood the test of time."

David Kibbe is based in New York City where he resides with his wife, the glamorous actress and author Susan Slavin, and the ghosts of their King Charles spaniels, Bliss and Passion.

For information about David Kibbe's work and products, visit: *www.davidkibbe.co.*

Hardback ISBN 978-0-593-58114-8
Ebook ISBN 978-0-593-58115-5

Printed in China

rodalebooks.com | randomhousebooks.com

2 4 6 8 9 7 5 3 1

First Edition

Book design by Headcase Design
Before and after photos by Maurizio Bacci – Babaldi Studio
Illustrations by Chandan Moharty

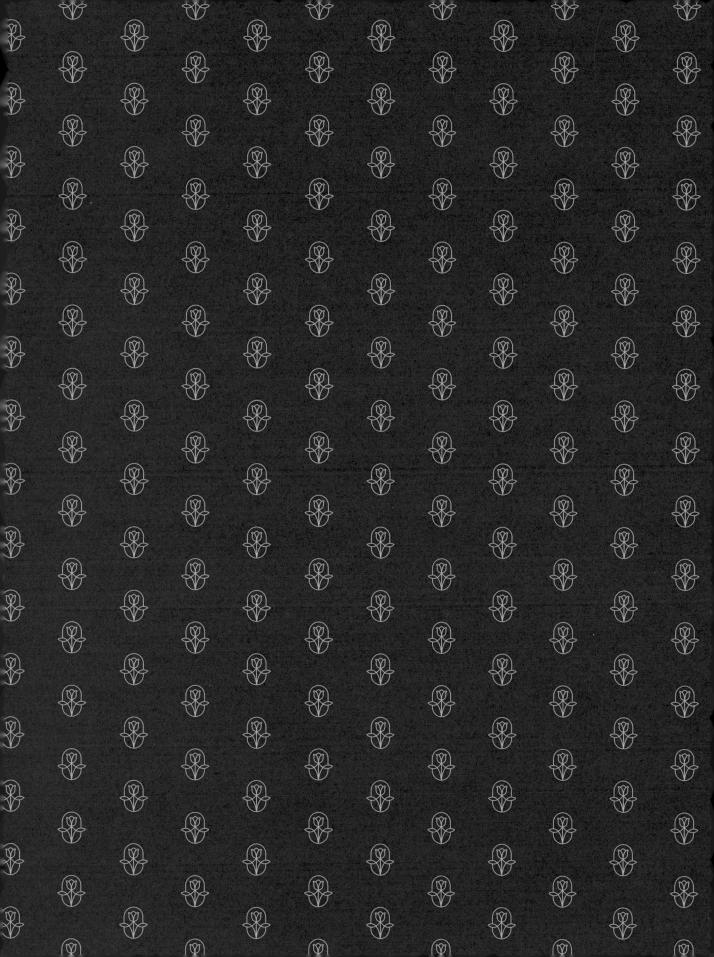

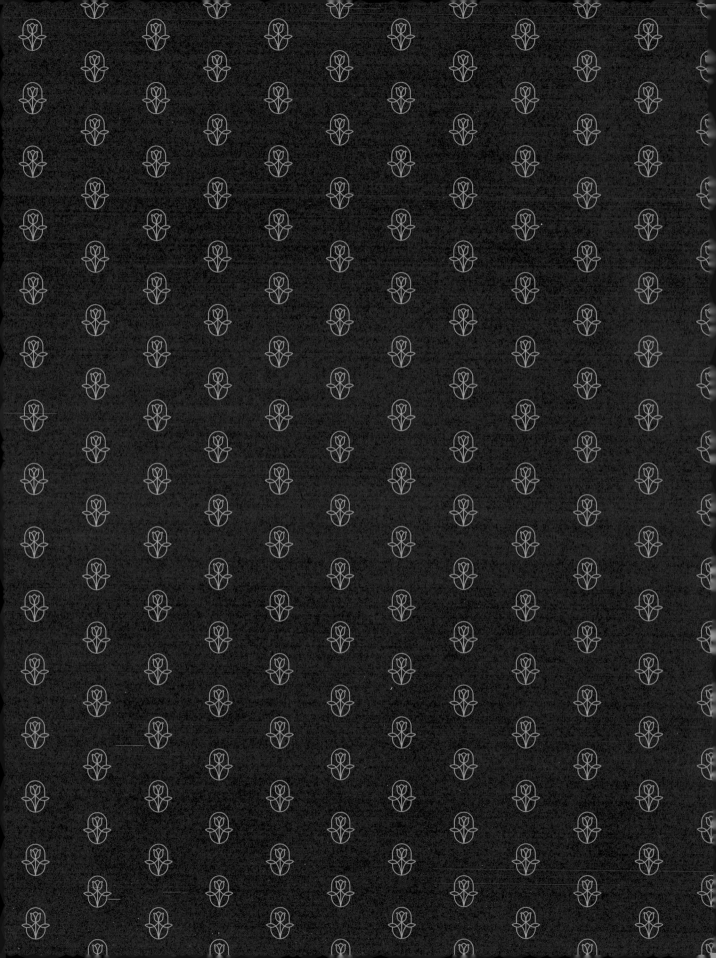